MUM'S WAY

Ian Millthorpe

with Lynne Barrett-Lee

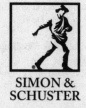

**SIMON &
SCHUSTER**

London · New York · Sydney · Toronto · New Delhi

A CBS COMPANY

First published in Great Britain by Simon & Schuster UK Ltd, 2013
A CBS COMPANY

1 3 5 7 9 10 8 6 4 2

Simon & Schuster UK Ltd
1st Floor
222 Gray's Inn Road
London WC1X 8HB

www.simonandschuster.co.uk

Simon & Schuster Australia,
Sydney

Simon & Schuster India,
New Delhi

A CIP catalogue record for this book is available from the British Library

ISBN: 978-1-47112-664-2
Ebook ISBN: 978-1-47112-665-9

Typeset in the UK by M Rules
Printed and bound by CPI Group (UK) Ltd, Croydon, CR0 4YY

I would like to dedicate this book to my beloved wife, Angie, and to the many wonderful mothers whose lives have been taken by cancer, and to remind them that, even after death, we still feel their love.

Chapter 1

March 2010

'Mill,' Angie calls to me. 'Come here a minute, will you?'

My name's Ian, but Angie has always called me Mill: Mill for Millthorpe – a shorter and more macho version of the school nickname I'd had the misfortune to have been saddled with, which couldn't have been worse: it was Milly.

I stop clearing away the breakfast things and go to see what she wants. Because that's what you do when your wife calls you, isn't it? It's a weekday and we're getting the younger kids ready for school. The youngest five of them, that is. Youngest five of the eight of them. Which means it's always something of a military operation in our house.

I go into the living room to find Angie plaiting our daughter Jade's hair in front of the mirror above the fireplace – something she's done every morning since Jade started school.

'Mill, stand here,' she says to me, beckoning me to the spot beside her. 'Just stand beside me and watch how I do this.'

She must have noticed my expression because she smiles at me then. 'It's easy when you know how,' she reassures me. 'It is, honest.'

I stand and watch her. Watch the way her hands move so swiftly and cleverly. 'I'll never be able to do that,' I say.

'Yes, you will,' Angie replies quietly. 'Because I'm going to teach you.'

Jade loves having her hair plaited. So she's almost in a trance. She's also, as usual, glued to a cartoon on TV, same as the rest of the little ones. 'Why d'you need to teach me?' I ask Angie, our eyes meeting their reflections in the mirror. Angie's looking so thin to me now. Even though she won't have it, and keeps telling me she's fine. Her own hair is back to normal now, since her last lot of chemo – just as full and soft and glossy as it's been since she was a teenager. But the rest of her seems to be shrinking before my eyes; she has to hoick her jeans up a hundred times a day now.

She stops plaiting Jade's hair for a moment and looks at me pointedly. 'Why?' I say again. 'Why d'you need to teach me, when you can do it?'

Now she gives me another little smile. Even the tiniest suggestion of one makes her whole face light up. 'You know why, Mill,' she says, in a voice that's now a whisper. 'Because one day you might have to do this yourself.'

I feel the tears begin to well in my eyes – tears I don't want anyone seeing. I don't want Angie to see them, and I don't want Jade to see them, either. So I just rush into the kitchen as quickly as I can. It's hard to stop myself crying, but I know I have to. Reece has already left for work, but, bar Jake, who I know has just gone upstairs to clean his teeth, all the other children are in the living room with Angie, and the last thing they need is to see their dad cry.

I'm having to do this so much now that I should be getting better at it, shouldn't I? And I suppose I sort of am. I get myself together, splash some water on my face to swill my tears away, then return to the living room, where Angie's now finished doing Jade's hair.

'Off you go,' she tells her. 'Go and get your shoes and your school bag.'

Then she turns and looks at me pointedly. 'Stop getting yourself all upset, Mill,' she tells me sternly. 'You're going to make yourself ill.' Her expression softens then. 'Look, love, I don't want to upset you, I really don't. But I need to know you're going to be okay.'

I can feel the tears threatening to start again and I know Angie can see it too. How can she stay so strong when I feel so overwhelmed?

'I need to know you're going to be able to look after the *kids*, Mill,' she says. 'Look, you take them to school, okay, and when we get back we need to have a little talk about this, okay?'

I nod dumbly at her, feeling humbled by her courage. My beautiful, beautiful wife, standing there in front of me and talking about what is going to happen to me after she dies. I don't know how I am going to bear it. Only that I have to.

Our middle three – Connor, and our twins, Jake and Jade – all go to the local school, Milefield Primary. Little Corey does as well – he does mornings at their nursery; has been going there since last September. And, as Angie's never driven, delivering them there is my job. Has been since I had to take early retirement in 2004, aged just forty-two, after having a brain haemorrhage.

The route to school is so familiar I could probably do it with my eyes closed. And, though I don't do it with my eyes closed, I definitely do it on autopilot, on the surface talking to Connor – being ten, he's in the front seat, and chattering away to me about something – but with my mind whirring with horrible, inescapable thoughts.

Normally, I wouldn't go straight home after dropping the children off. Angie's mum and dad live just a little way down the street from us, and I usually stop by to say hello on my return journey, just to see if there's anything they need doing. They're getting on now, Herbert and Winnie, and Winnie's quite frail, so I tend to do any heavy stuff that needs doing, run errands for them, that kind of thing. But today I don't. Today I drive straight back home, heart in mouth, anxious to get back to Angie.

When I get indoors, she's dusting in the living room, so I go into the kitchen to make us both a cup of tea, then take it in and sit down on the sofa. 'Okay, Angie,' I say, trying to keep my voice level as she sits down. 'What's on your mind, love?'

She puts her mug of tea down and takes my hand.

'Mill,' she says. 'I've been thinking, okay? I need to know that if – *when* – anything happens to me, that you and the kids will be okay.'

'Stop worrying,' I say. Because that's what you always say, isn't it? Even though we both know it's no longer a case of 'if'. Not any more. Now it's just a case of 'when'. 'We'll manage,' I add. 'We *will*. We'll be okay.'

I can hardly deal with even thinking about it, to be honest. So I try not to. But Angie is having none of it. 'Can you plait the girls' hair?' she asks, smiling at me.

'No,' I say. 'You know I can't. And I don't know any man who can, either.'

She's stopped smiling now, and I can see that she's struggling with what she wants to say to me just as much as I am with having to hear it. 'Mill,' she says. 'I know that. But you're going to be different from most men. Most men don't have to be Mum as well as Dad, do they? But you're going to. That's what you'll *have* to be.'

I put my arms round her and hold her tight. There's no one to see now, and she's crying too. The tears are rolling in streams down her face. 'We'll be okay, Angie, love,' I reassure her. 'I promise.'

She pulls back slightly to look at me, wiping her tears with the back of her hand. 'But it's going to be so *hard*. That's all I keep thinking about. All our babies ... the logistics of it all ... it's all going to be so *hard* for you. So I've been thinking, and I need to make it as easy as I can for you. I'm going to *show* you.' She sniffs her remaining tears away. She means business, suddenly. I can see it by the look in her eyes. I know that look well. Angie's never been one for giving up. You don't have eight kids if you're one for giving up. 'I'm going to teach you everything,' she says. 'I'm going to make sure you know everything you need to know, from bathing them to feeding them, to helping them with their homework, to ... to ... yes, to baking cakes. You *have* to know how to do that, Mill. That's important.'

'Baking cakes?' I can't see myself learning how to bake *any-thing*.

'Yes. For the kids' *birthdays*,' she says, looking at me as if I should have known that already. And as she speaks I can see that she *has* thought about this. That she really does need reassuring that we'll manage without her. That I can whip up a birthday cake, at the very least.

'Okay, love,' I say. I'm really just so grateful to see her smile again. 'Tell me, then. When do I start?'

I suppose everyone likes to think that their first love will be their only love, especially when you find yourself first falling in love at the impressionable and tender age of fourteen. But how often does that happen? Hardly ever.

The 27th of September 1976 is a date I will never forget. It was late afternoon and I was walking home from my mate David's house, when I heard someone call to me from across the road. I looked up to see a girl I knew from school running across to me. 'Ian,' she said breathlessly, 'will you go on a date with my mate, Angie? She really fancies you,' she added by way of enticement.

I said no. I desperately wanted to say yes but I said no. I'd seen Angie around and I really fancied her as well, but I was fourteen and I was sceptical because I knew what girls were like. It was a joke, I decided. Had to be. I could imagine saying yes, and then this girl running back and telling Angie, and then both of them having a good laugh at my expense.

Plus, it was raining now, raining hard, and I didn't want to hang around getting wet. This was the seventies, so I had my

6

hair to think of. 'Oh, *go* on, Ian,' she pleaded. '*Seriously*. She really, *really* likes you! She's always talking about you,' she added. 'Go on. *Please*?'

I was still uncertain, obviously, because I still wasn't convinced it wasn't some sort of windup, but I decided I should chance it even so. I really did fancy Angie Yoxall, after all. And if I said no – well, I might miss my chance, mightn't I? She was really pretty, too – with those enormous brown eyes of hers – so suppose someone else snapped her up instead? 'Okay,' I said, trying to sound as cool as I could manage. 'Tell her I'll meet her at the park after school tomorrow. Six o'clock.'

The park was close to the school, and a few of us liked to hang out there. It had all the usual things – a bowling green, tennis courts, a then derelict pavilion. Plus plenty of benches on which to while away a sunny afternoon with a girl. If you had one . . .

The girl, who was also called Angie, ran off satisfied, saying she'd let the other Angie know, and I carried on home, grinning from ear to ear. I couldn't believe it. My first date! My first date *ever*! I had a girlfriend! That was how it worked then; none of this long-winded stuff kids do on Facebook these days. I had a date, which meant I had a girlfriend – well, more or less. I didn't care about the rain now, even though I was getting completely drenched. The next day couldn't come soon enough.

Or go quickly enough, either, once I got to it. First loves are an all-consuming business, and I could hardly concentrate on anything. I was too obsessed with trying to catch a glimpse of Angie. I'd see her around all the time normally –

couldn't miss her, because I fancied her – but today she was frustratingly elusive. Break time, then lunchtime, then second break came around. And not a sign of her. Was she even *in* school today?

And then, as I left for home, there she was, by the school gates. And she was clearly waiting for me, I realised – I could tell by the way she looked up as I approached. And, as I tried to walk up looking as nonchalant as possible, she peeled away from the wall by the school gates that she'd been leaning on, and strolled up to me, a blur of huge eyes and chocolate-coloured hair.

'Hi, Milly,' she said shyly. I loved her shyness. 'I was just wondering. Can we meet at five instead of six?'

She waited for my answer, offering no explanation for the time change. 'Sure,' I said, still trying to avoid sounding even remotely eager. To sound too eager was the worst thing you could *ever* do. 'That's okay with me,' I added. 'See you at five instead, then.'

'Thanks,' she said. And then she was gone.

I walked home on air for the second day running, my smile widening with every step I took. Blimey, I thought, with typically simple teenage logic. Can't even wait till six o'clock to meet me – she must really like me! I walked faster. I had a lot to do between now and five o'clock.

I was in the front door, bag dumped, and up the stairs like a rocket. First up was a bath, and, while that was running, a decision about what I should wear. After a quick rummage through my wardrobe – accompanied by a backing track of David Bowie – I shot back down to Mum with my best trousers. They were beige and high-waisted, with big pockets and two rows of buttons. They were the coolest things I owned, bar my cherry-red Doc Martens, which I would naturally be wearing as well. 'Mum,' I said, smiling sweetly at her. 'Do you think you can run the iron over these for me?'

I was the youngest of eight kids (my closest brother, Glenn, was eighteen now) and, because I was the baby of the family, Mum spoilt me rotten. Sometimes, if I was going out, she'd even follow me with change in her pocket, so she could give it to me without the others seeing. I don't think they'd have minded, though. She spoilt us all, really. And as by now there were just three of my brothers, Terry, Les and Glenn, at home, she had a bit more time on her hands than she used to.

She smiled, as she always did, and held her arm out to take the trousers. 'You're in a hurry, lad,' she observed. 'You got yourself a woman?'

I felt a blush shoot up my cheeks. It just kind of exploded there. I couldn't stop it. 'No,' I said quickly. 'I'm just going round my mate's house.'

'Of course you are,' I heard her answer as I headed back upstairs to have my bath.

I didn't have much time to sit in the tub and consider my good fortune, however, as the clock was ticking steadily towards five now. There was just time to dry myself, grab the trousers (trying to pretend I hadn't noticed Mum's amused expression) and as an afterthought – I was halfway up the garden path when it occurred to me – to go back and nip into Terry's room and pinch a splash or two of his Brut aftershave. It was vital that I not only look my best for Angie but

9

that I smell my best as well. He'd kill me if he knew, but, all being well, he wouldn't. And, if he suspected, I'd just deny everything, anyway. A man had to do what a man had to do, after all. In this case 'splash it on', just as the boxer Henry Cooper told me in the TV ads.

I half walked and half ran down the slumbering late-afternoon streets, and, with the aftershave scenting the air in my wake, I was at Grimethorpe Park, ready for my date, on the dot of five.

They talk about your heart skipping a beat and all that mushy stuff, but I'm sure that, when I clapped eyes on Angie, mine did. Two or three beats, in fact, because sitting there, on the nearest bench, the one just inside the park gates, she looked more beautiful than ever. The flower beds were bare now, stripped of all their summer marigolds and geraniums. But, even if they hadn't been, no flower could have matched up to her. She looked perfect. Too good to be true.

'Hi,' she said. And, if anything, she looked even shyer than she had before.

'Hi,' I said, sitting down on the bench beside her. I took in faded denim jeans, a cream jumper – the fluffy sort, hand-knitted, looked like – and that tumble of sheeny chocolate hair. I couldn't take my eyes off her. She had the most amazing smile, ever, and I'm pretty certain I fell in love with her that very day.

I couldn't believe my luck. I never could. I still can't. She was my first love *and* my only. And my last.

Chapter 2

Learning to plait hair was never going to be something that came easily to me. I dare say there are men out there who learnt it at their mother's knee, but I definitely wasn't one of them. I come from a traditional mining family, based in the village of Grimethorpe, near Barnsley, where plaiting hair isn't high on most men's agendas.

Grimethorpe is probably best known for coalmining, the two pits there being among the deepest in Britain. Up till the pits closed, almost half the population worked in the mining industry, and when all that finished, as well as half the population being unemployed, there were, and still are, lots of disabled people living here, as a legacy of all those years working underground.

Though there are no longer any working mines, Grimethorpe is still a close-knit mining community, and, like many others in South Yorkshire, it's almost as famous – perhaps more so – for its colliery brass band. But, as depicted in the 1996 film *Brassed Off*, which was also filmed here, there were some years of real struggle after the pit closures. In fact the plot is based on what happened to the real colliery band at that time. Happily, however, the band thrives to this day, and even performed at the London 2012 Olympics.

The village and its people also have another claim to fame, though, because a close family friend (and former miner), Freddie Fletcher, had a leading role in the 1969 film, *Kes*. And the world that film depicted really hasn't changed that much. The landscape may have altered, but the people definitely haven't – there's still the same sense of belonging, the sense of community. And the big sprawling intertwined families.

As a fourteen-year-old in the 1970s, I certainly knew where my future career lay: I would follow my father and train as a miner at Grimethorpe Colliery. Like most of my contemporaries, I was very proud to do so.

But all thoughts of the future disappeared from my mind on the day Angie Yoxall agreed to be my girlfriend. Time, on that day, seemed to stop altogether.

'Oh, God, Mill – look at the time!' she said, rising from the park bench. Somehow, nearly five hours had passed without either of us noticing. It was pitch dark, freezing cold, and she was supposed to be back by ten.

'I'll walk you home,' I offered gallantly, even though I had no idea where she lived. And, as a reward for my chivalry, Angie let me kiss her goodnight. That was it, for me, that kiss. I knew, floating home, that I was done for.

We fell in love swiftly, as teenagers do. Within weeks there was hardly a wall anywhere in Grimethorpe that one or other of us hadn't chalked our names on. We saw each other almost every day, meeting up in school, in the playground, and then dashing out to meet again after school, for our five o'clock tryst in the park.

By now, as the winter was beginning to bite, we had graduated from the bench near the park entrance to a step that led up to the derelict pavilion – or, rather, '*our* step', as Angie soon christened it.

Looking back, I'm amazed we didn't perish in the bitter cold, as we'd spend hours and hours sitting there, huddled close together on the cold concrete, talking about everything and nothing, as you do. But somehow we didn't seem to feel the harsh Yorkshire winter – perhaps love really does keep you warm.

Naturally, I was terrified at the prospect of meeting Angie's parents, assuming, as I imagine most teenage boys probably do, that I wouldn't be good enough for their daughter. But her dad, it turned out, was a retired collier, as mine was, and had worked with my dad for many years.

His name was Herbert, and he couldn't have been friendlier. 'A know your dad, lad,' he said, in his broad Yorkshire accent. 'Used to work with him down the pit. Lovely fella.'

Which seemed to mean I was accepted into their family, which was a massive relief. And, from that day, he and Winnie – who would become like a second mum to me – treated me as one of their own children. So now, though we'd still meet at the park on school days and at weekends, I'd be up out of bed and out calling on Angie before she could even wipe the sleep out of her eyes.

For all that, for some reason, she didn't seem to tire of me, and the weeks turned to months, which became years. 'Together forever', we used to say. And we meant it. If there was a more perfect girl in Yorkshire, I didn't reckon I'd ever find her. I already had. Angie and I were for keeps.

We both left school in the summer of 1978. I wanted to be a miner, like my dad, so, once I was accepted, I followed family tradition and began working in the colliery, doing my initial surface training. Angie had always been keen on getting a job working with children, so she was thrilled to begin a six-month training course at the local nursery. It was her dream job; once she started, those kids were all she ever talked about. How their little faces would light up when she sat and read them a story, and how much joy taking care of them gave her. So it was no surprise that almost the first thing she said to me on our wedding night a few years later was, 'Can we start a family right away?'

And I was no less keen than she was – this was our honeymoon, after all, so I was understandably enthusiastic about trying, even if we did have to spend a considerable time beforehand clearing our hotel bed of all the rice her brother Neil had sneaked up and put in there. And her wedding-night wish was granted, as well. Two months later she came home waving a small brown envelope from the chemist's: the result for the sample she'd dropped in there a few days back.

'So,' she said gleefully. 'What d'you reckon, Mill? Am I or aren't I?'

And, to my great pride – in a job pretty well done, I reckoned – the piece of paper confirmed that she was.

You couldn't move then, in our house, for baby things. At this time we were living in our first proper home, a three-bed semi in the village of Shafton, just two miles from Grimethorpe, and right away it was all about planning for the baby. We did up a nursery with white clouds, a blue sky and a rainbow, and Angie pored over every baby magazine going. She really couldn't wait to be a mum, because it was all she really wanted: to spend her life surrounded by kids. There was sadness as well as happiness in our lives then, however. Tragically, my poor dad wasn't around to welcome his youngest grandchild into the world. Like so many miners, he'd paid the ultimate price for his years of hard and dangerous work, and the coal dust he'd inhaled for over forty-five years was, at the age of sixty-eight, about to end his life.

But Angie said her goodbyes to him in her usual special way. Saying farewell on what would turn out to be the second-to-last day of his life, she didn't cry – instead she gave him a big kiss on his cheek, then reached out and grabbed hold of his big, sticky-out ears. She then burst out laughing. And Angie's laugh was really something.

'You know,' she said, grinning, 'I've always wanted to get hold of those big lugs and squash 'em!' Which brought a smile to Dad's face as well as a tear to his eye.

'Come here, love,' he said, pulling her closer by the bedside, so he could stroke her swollen belly and say goodbye to the grandchild he'd never see. And I remember thinking just how amazing my wife was.

*

Our first child, Ryan Arthur, was born just a little over a month later, and I remember it as well as if I'd given birth to him myself. I know most men are pretty feeble compared with women when it comes to pain, but, when our son began showing signs that he was about to join the family, I'm pretty sure I felt every contraction along with Angie.

And it was no wonder that I probably screamed louder than she did. Because Angie – being told to '*push!*' – obviously needed something to grip onto, and, since my head was handy (I was at the head end rather than the business end), it seemed to make sense to her to grab hold of my hair, with both hands. Fortunately, it wasn't too extended a labour, or I'd probably still be bald to this day.

As it was, once we were done, and Ryan was safely with us, all Angie could do was burst out laughing. I had scratches down my face and whole clumps of hair missing. I looked as if I'd fought a lion and lost.

Once home, Angie could barely bring herself to put our baby son down. While my flesh wounds healed up and my hair started regrowing, she would sit for hours nursing him, relishing every precious moment and, whenever I watched the pair of them, despite the ordeal I'd had to go through to get here, I really thought I'd burst with love and pride.

And it wasn't too long before we tried for another, because Angie wasn't content to stop at one. And neither was I. We were both of us from big families – that was what we were used to.

'I'd love a girl this time,' Angie said. 'So I can dress her up and plait her hair, and, when she's older, the pair of us can go clothes shopping together, and then, one day, I'll see her in a beautiful white wedding dress, walking up the aisle.'

It was the same dream any mum would have, so why wouldn't she dream that? But, when Damon arrived, Angie couldn't have cared less. Once again, she was like a little girl with a new doll to play with; she just loved babies, and nothing about caring for them seemed to faze her. She just seemed born to do it, doing what she was meant to.

And, unsurprisingly, it didn't take much longer for her to whistle up number three. And when Reece came along, in the spring of 1991, she positively whooped with delight. With two mini-Mills running around (well, one running, one careering around, mostly crashing into furniture), she was thrilled to see Reece's shock of inky hair and olive skin. 'At last!' she cried. 'I have one that looks a little bit like me!'

Not that life was quite like something off *The Waltons*. Though Angie had a part-time job as a cleaner at the high school just behind our house, with three kids to feed, money was the tightest it had ever been and my eight-hour dark and dusty shifts down the mine were now regularly stretching to twelve. I didn't care, though. I had what I wanted. Where once my definition of happiness would have been me and Angie on the road in my Mark 1 blue Capri, I now measured happiness differently. I felt blessed. I had Angie. I had my boys. And I had a life filled with love. Everything I knew I'd *ever* want.

But fate, it seemed, had other plans for us. Plans that became evident one blustery Saturday in March 1993. I was sitting on the sofa nursing Reece at the time. He was getting on for two now and we called him Mr Mischief. You couldn't leave him five minutes in the vicinity of a kitchen cupboard without him pulling every last pot and pan out over the floor.

Angie walked in with an odd sort of look on her face. It was a worried look and, as Angie was someone who spent most of her life smiling, it was an expression I didn't often see.

'Mill,' she said. 'I think I've found a lump in my breast.'

I put Reece down as she unbuttoned her blouse to show me. 'There, look,' she said, taking my hand to guide me to it. 'Can you feel it?'

I could. There was a definite lump there, but it felt tiny. No bigger than the size of a pea. 'I don't think that's anything to worry about,' I told her. 'It's very small. It's probably just a cyst. But better be safe than sorry. Let's make an appointment at the doctor's. Though I'm sure it's nothing to worry about,' I said again.

And that was what we kept saying, right up till we went to the appointment, because at that time what else would we think? Angie was only thirty. Whoever heard of women getting breast cancer at thirty? Not us, for sure. It just didn't seem possible.

The GP agreed we were probably right not to worry. 'It certainly feels like it could be a cyst,' she confirmed. 'But I'll refer you to the hospital for a biopsy, anyway, just to make sure.'

The biopsy done, it was a couple of weeks later that we got

the letter in the post asking Angie to attend the clinic for her results. And we were still neither of us that worried, not really. It was such a tiny lump, she was so young, and there was no cancer in any of her family, after all.

'Don't be daft, Mill,' she said to me, when I told her I'd take the day off to take her. Angie didn't drive so it would be easiest if I took her. But she was insistent. 'There's no need, honest, Mill. I'll ask Mam to go with me.'

'Are you sure?' I said. Though it would be difficult to get a shift off now that I was working at the colliery in Pontefract, I still felt it was my responsibility to be with her.

'No, Mill,' she said firmly. 'You go to work. Don't take a day off just for this. I'll go with Mam. And stop worrying, will you? I'll be *fine*.'

I couldn't think of anything but Angie all day. Didn't matter how much we'd convinced ourselves there was nothing seriously wrong with her, I just couldn't help thinking, 'Yes, but what if there is?'

And, when I got home from work, it was to find the doors locked and the house empty, which meant the boys must be still round my mum's. I felt a cold chill begin to creep up my spine. It was two thirty in the afternoon now, and Angie's appointment at the hospital had been at ten. So where the hell was she? She should have been back ages ago.

Really worried now, and not knowing whether to go up the road to Mum's or wait at home for Angie, I ended up pacing the living room, looking out of the front window for a glimpse of her, every minute of waiting feeling like half an hour.

In fact, it was a full hour before I finally caught sight of her in the distance, walking slowly and stiffly up the street. Everything in her gait felt all wrong – so not like Angie. I think I knew even then that it was going to be bad news. I ran to the front door and opened it, and, even at a distance, I could see from her expression that something *was* badly wrong. My heart seemed to plummet to my boots.

As she got to the gate, she finally saw me, and looked at me, shaking her head. She was crying. I ran down the path and pulled her close to me, trying to brace myself for what was coming.

Our happy little bubble was about to be burst. 'I've got cancer,' she sobbed into my chest.

Chapter 3

To my relief, because I'm so addled that I'm all fingers and thumbs now, we don't have another hair-plaiting lesson then and there. The kids are all in school now – Jade obviously included – and, in any case, the household chores won't do themselves.

So Angie, who has now dried her eyes and seems to be in determined mood again, has another idea. Ella Rose is down for her nap on the sofa in the living room, so, while she sleeps, we're going to continue with some cooking.

'Chicken curry,' Angie decides, once we're back in the kitchen and she's inspecting the contents of the freezer. 'You can help me make the kids' favourite chicken curry for tea.'

Having decided we have everything we need in terms of ingredients, she starts pulling utensils from drawers. I watch her. Watch the way she moves so purposefully around the kitchen. A chopping board, a couple of knives, a saucepan, and then another. It's as if she were the captain of a ship and I some hopeless new recruit.

We've been twenty-three years in this house – we moved in when Ryan was a baby – and we decorated it together, working every spare hour in the evenings and on the weekends, spending days and days stripping wallpaper. Then chose new stuff – though it took forever, because we could never agree on anything. If Angie liked it, I didn't, and vice versa, every time. Though, naturally, the house ended up decorated to her specifications. Where our home was concerned, it was always Angie's way from the word go.

'Come on, you,' she says now, pointing to a pile of onions on the worktop. 'It won't make itself. Go on. Get chopping!'

I'm not stupid. I can attack a vegetable that needs peeling as well as the next man, but like most men – certainly men doing the twelve-hour shifts underground that I used to – up to now I haven't encountered a lot of veg that does. Haven't encountered a lot of veg that needs peeling, full stop.

Back in the day, when I was still working in the collieries, I was a tunneller. I was one of a team of four men, and two of the others, Danny and John, I'd been friends with all my life. We'd work straight twelve-hour shifts, stopping only to eat the packed lunch we'd taken down with us, and take it in turns to drive the machine. It was a massive brute of a thing, called a Dosco Roadheader, which would cut through the rock and coal, a metre at a time, and then we'd carry large RSJs (rolled steel joists, which were hefty girders) to build the framework of the tunnel we'd just created. We'd bolt it together on the floor of the tunnel and then use the Roadheader's long cutting boom to lift the finished section of new frame into position.

It was heavy work. Sometimes we'd have to carry the girders – just the four of us – for anything up to thirty metres, sometimes up to our knees in sludge and mud. But we'd never slacken – we didn't dare to. My older brother Barry was our foreman, and very keen as well. If he felt anyone wasn't doing the job right, he'd report them to the manager, and he showed no favouritism towards his little brother. He had a couple of nicknames, as well, which I still rib him about now: Barry the Bastard and the Laughing Assassin. But, for all that, it was a great working atmosphere down there, and his being a stickler didn't seem to reduce his popularity any; everybody seemed to like our Barry.

It was extremely hot work. And, whatever the weather on the surface, it was always humid underground, and we'd be sweltering. So every day we'd wear nothing else but boots, shorts and helmets, and one of the essentials was a large water bottle that you'd take down full of ice cubes, so that at least you'd have something cold to drink. We'd come up again black. Black to the pore, just as you'd expect. Blacker than the coal itself, we always used to say.

As I stand in my kitchen now, chopping onions while my wife gives me instructions, it suddenly seems a very long time ago. But I'm prepared to learn. Because my life is different now, and one day I know it's going to change even more. And, though even thinking about being without Angie upsets me to distraction, I'm prepared to work hard to learn the things she wants to teach me. Painful though it is to con-template why I'm learning all these skills, I want to give her the peace of mind I know she needs now.

Ella's just woken up crying, so, while Angie goes to see to her, I begin chopping the onions she's given me. Our two dogs, Jess and Pebbles, keep an eye on my every move – just in case something edible might come their way. Bits of chicken, raw onion – they're not fussy. And then I stop, the onions done. Which is my first mistake, apparently. Because as soon as Angie comes back in, Ella in her arms, to see how I'm getting on, she immediately laughs her big booming laugh.

It hasn't diminished, Angie's laugh. Not a bit. 'Not like that!' she admonishes. 'You need to chop it smaller! The kids won't touch it if it's in those great galumphing lumps. Here,' she says, handing me Ella, so she can demonstrate. 'You need to cut it up much finer. Look. See what I do, okay?' She grabs another onion, and, after peeling it, shows me how to cut it crossways so I can easily chop it into much smaller dice. And as she does so I realise just how thin her wrists have got now. How much less there is of her now, full stop.

I let her help me long enough to get the hang of it, then wrestle the vegetable knife back off her. And, sure enough, the more I chop, the more the onions start to get to me and within minutes I'm unable to stem the flow of tears that are rolling down my face.

I don't try to stop them. Why would I? They provide cover for the real reason I'm standing here crying. Because it's not the onions themselves that are making my eyes water: it's that, while I chop them up and transform them into tiny glistening pieces, I get a picture in my mind that I just can't shake off. It's of me again, standing here, just as I am now, in our kitchen. And everything's the same as it is at this moment. I'm chopping onions to make the kids their special chicken curry, Ella's close by – perhaps sitting in her high chair with a cup of juice – and the dogs are hovering hopefully, just the way they have been today, looking up at me with bug expectant eyes, waiting for morsels. Only when it's made – when I've made Angie's special chicken curry, all by myself – I'm going to be serving it with an empty place at the table.

On hearing the word 'cancer' that day back in 1993, it felt like a knife was going through me. It just seemed too incredible to be true. How could Angie have cancer at her age? I just couldn't believe it.

But she had. Against all the odds, she had the killer disease – the disease that terrified absolutely everyone it touched. And I was no exception. The thought of losing her just seemed to stop my heart. I didn't know what to say to her, what to do, how to help her. I just held her as tightly as I could.

It was spring and the front garden was already looking lovely. Like almost everyone in my family, I was a very keen gardener at that time, and, as well as growing as much as I could from seed in my greenhouse, I spent lots of my spare time outdoors, working on it. We had a perfect striped lawn, which I had always been so proud of, and already the beds and baskets were full of pansies and primroses, which would soon be replaced with flowers for summer. Suddenly it meant nothing. Suddenly the world felt dark. Hearing those words leached the colour out of everything.

'I've got breast cancer, Mill,' Angie said again, into my

chest. The tears were running freely down her cheeks as she clutched me and sobbed. 'I can't believe it. I just can't believe it.'

'Come on,' I said, coaxing her back up the path. It must have felt like the longest journey home ever, and I felt so angry with myself that I hadn't insisted on going with her. Even angrier with myself that I'd been so confident it wouldn't be this. That I was so completely unprepared for it. 'Come on,' I said. 'Let's get you back inside, in the warm.' Not that it was that cold. But it suddenly felt it. 'It'll be okay, love,' I reassured her. 'I know it will. They can cure breast cancer these days. And they've caught it early, haven't they? So I'm sure they'll be able to get rid of it.'

'Mill, I can't believe it,' she said again. 'I've got *breast cancer*.'

And she would have to have her breast removed. That was the next thing she told me, once I'd got her inside and we'd sat down on the sofa. She'd already gone in with her mum, she said, and told her dad. I knew they would be as shocked as I was. She was just so *young*.

'That doesn't matter,' I said. And, even as I said that, it felt all wrong. Of course it mattered that she'd lose her breast. It would matter to *her* – I knew it would. But she had to know it wouldn't matter to *me*. That it wouldn't change anything between us. 'All that matters is that you get better,' I said. 'That you're going to be all right. That's all I care about.'

Everything seemed to happen really quickly after that, which only increased the feeling that this was something very serious. Angie was given a date for her mastectomy, after which, they explained, she would be given a course of radiotherapy, which – assuming all was well, as far as they could tell, anyway – would be the end of it and we could get on with our lives.

That date couldn't come soon enough. Now we knew it was there, we just couldn't stop thinking about it. Imagining the cancer that was lurking inside Angie's body – lurking *and* growing. How fast *could* it grow? Even though we'd been reassured by the oncologist that the outcome looked positive, every day we waited seemed one too many. But the days passed, and, on a hot, sunny Tuesday at the beginning of July, I took her into Barnsley Hospital to have her operation the following day. Now it was imminent, I felt happier, knowing it would soon be gone from her body, and, by now, my main concern anyway was that I needed to reassure her that I didn't care that she'd come out minus one breast. She was hard to convince that I wouldn't react badly to seeing her scar, but nothing could have been further from the truth. All I cared about was that she get well again.

I went to see Angie after her op with mixed emotions. On the one hand I was so relieved to know that the cancer had been taken away, but, on the other, a mastectomy must have felt like such a brutal thing to go through, and I thought she'd be really upset.

I dropped Ryan at school, and then took Damon and Reece round to my brother Malc's house, reflecting that it already felt as if I'd done a day's work, just getting them all up and dressed and fed.

Angie's brother Neil and his wife Diane came with me. Neil was the closest in age to Angie (he was three years her senior and they also shared a birthday) and, over the years since Angie and I had got together, the four of us had become really close. They had two kids, Lee and Jane, now eleven and eight respectively, and, before we had our own kids, wherever we went, little Lee would always be on my shoulders. We did a lot together, the four of us – we were always in each other's houses – and every year, when the whole family went away to Rhyl together, it was invariably the four of us who were up to mischief. In fact, 'mischief' doesn't cover it: we were professionals.

Our finest hour, perhaps, was back in our early years as a couple, not long after the two families had started going away on holiday together. We'd been joining Angie's lot for two weeks in Rhyl for a couple of years now, not just me and Angie, but half my siblings as well, plus their other halves, Les and Glenn, and, now Dad had died, our mum too. We really were like one enormous happy family. And, on this particular holiday, we were up to our tricks as usual, having bought some farting powder from a joke shop on the front.

We loved going to the joke shop – I think everyone loved visiting seaside joke shops back in those days – and would regularly play tricks on each other. We loved getting those little bits of foil you could stick in the tops of cigarettes, which exploded when the unlucky recipient tried to light them, and the ones that made your fag smell like burning rubber. We also loved that soap you could get that turned your face black when you washed with it – I even managed to get Angie with that one, one holiday. Sad to think no one would fall for it now.

That particular night everyone went out to the pub across the road from the flats we were staying in, and, as Winnie was the target of our mischief that evening, every time she left the table, Neil and I spiked her drink with the farting powder. And, as waiting for something to happen is almost as much fun as if and when it *does* happen, Angie and Diane were in tears almost, from having to stifle giggles every time their eyes met across the table.

But nothing did happen, and Winnie left the pub as she'd entered it, oblivious and (as far as we knew) flatulence-free, and we all agreed that, though the powder had been a bit of a disappointment, we'd been in such stitches waiting for something explosive to happen, it was probably worth the price for that alone.

But the night wasn't over. Not just yet.

'Hey, you lot,' Herbert whispered as he put the key in the door to the flats. 'Don't you be making a noise when you get in there. Quiet as you go up them stairs, you hear? There's people trying to sleep, so you just keep it down.'

We were all of us a bit merry now, but we promised him we would, and carefully began making our way upstairs, behind him and Winnie, treading carefully so as not to make them creak. And we made it. We'd just reached our landing – in complete silence – when it happened: Winnie finally broke wind.

And impressively loudly, as well. 'Winnie!' hissed Herbert,

turning around to glare at her. 'Be *quiet*!' We exchanged looks, desperately trying to keep our faces straight as we did so. But it was Winnie herself who was our downfall. Once she started giggling there was no hope for any of us, and, to Herbert's disgust, we were soon all of us doubled up from trying to keep quiet, which could only lead to one inevitable conclusion: Angie would start properly laughing, and then we'd all be done for.

And she did. But it was poor Winnie who took the flak for that too. 'Look what you've done now, woman! You've only gone and set our Angie off! With that laugh of hers she'll wake the whole bloody street up!'

Needless to say, we never confessed.

We were none of us expecting Angie to be laughing much today; we'd have to do our very best to cheer her up. 'One of those'll do the trick,' said Neil now, as we passed the hospital shop. He was pointing to a blue helium balloon with the words GET WELL SOON on it. And, sure enough, when we got to the ward, as soon as Angie saw it, she just burst out laughing.

'Look at him with that big silly balloon,' she said, as he tied it to the end of her bed. 'You're crackers, Neil!' she said, clutching her chest theatrically. 'You'll have my stitches out!'

I could hardly believe how well she seemed. Yes, she looked tired, and she must surely have been in pain. And there was no escaping the fact that she wasn't even thirty-one years old, and had just had an operation to remove her breast. But her laughter reverberated round the whole ward, it was so infectious, and soon the other five women in there were laughing with us.

'Oh, I wish I had a bit of what she's got!' said the lady in the bed next to her. 'She *never* stops laughing. Have you put something in her water?'

I felt so proud of her that day.

Looking back, I think it was probably also on that day that I got taught my first lesson about just what an amazing job Angie did as well. Feeling much better now I'd seen her, I dropped Neil and Diane home, and picked the boys up from Malc and Eileen's in a much brighter frame of mind. We could none of us quite believe how well she seemed to be taking it. And, though we all agreed it would probably hit her a bit more once she started the radiotherapy, we were all just so pleased by how well she was coping.

A great deal better, it turned out, than I seemed to be myself. Because I could hardly cook back then (I'd never needed to: that was Angie's department), it was obviously going to be a struggle for a few days, and I knew my mam would help me out with some dinners, as would Malc and Eileen. But today it was just me and the boys, and they all needed feeding, and I decided I'd make them something even *I* couldn't mess up. Beans on toast all round, I thought. That would do.

But how *did* Angie do it, with three little boys in the house? Within minutes of our getting home, the whole house seemed in uproar. The sink was overflowing with dishes from where I'd left them that morning; there was mud all over the carpet from where Ryan and Damon had been running round the garden; and, with Reece being two and into everything he shouldn't be, I needed eyes in the back of my head.

And as I flapped around, trying to stir the beans, watch the toast, lay the table and get the drinks, I had all three boys tugging endlessly at my trouser leg.

'Dad, can we have an ice cream?'

'Dad, will you read us a story?'

'Dad, is dinner ready yet?'

'Dad, I'm hungry.'

'Dad, I'm thirsty.'

'Dad, I need the toilet.'

'Dad, I want you to play with me.'

'Dad, Reece has just pulled all the potatoes out of the veg rack!'

'Da-aadddd! Ryan hit me!'

'Da-aadddd! It were Damon!'

'*Dad*! When is Mum coming *home*?'

Soon, I hoped. *Soon*. Because I was already floundering. The house was in chaos, and I didn't know where to start. How could you ever start *anything* with three boys running around? And, even if you did start, how on earth did you finish?

I was in awe, as well as meltdown. It was all I could do just to get through the next half-dozen hours without one or the other of them ending up in Casualty or burning the house down. And, once I'd got them into bed, I was so tired that, when I finally sat down to watch telly, I immediately fell fast asleep.

My twelve-hour shifts at the coal mine didn't seem quite so hard any more, not compared with this. How on earth did Angie do it and still be smiling?

Chapter 4

Angie seems determined to turn me into some sort of master chef, because, a couple of weeks (and a couple of frustrating plaiting lessons) later, she decides I need to make a start on mastering the art of baking.

I'm sure training me up isn't all it's about, either, because when she comes into the living room the first thing her gaze rests on is the laptop. And I know why: it's because I'm sitting at it, as I so often am now, searching for ways to stop her dying. It's something that seems to take up a lot of my time now; it's taken over from almost everything else. I'm no longer working – not since I left the colliery in 2004 – but I've always had things on the go. Looking after Angie's parents, doing bits of decorating, taking Mum down to the shops, running the kids around, taking them to the park. And, back when we still had them, flying our Harris hawks. And of course the garden. I've completely lost interest in the garden this year. I keep the grass cut, front and back, so it looks tidy, but that's all.

It just feels as if there are only two things that matter at the moment: spending time with Angie, because we don't know how much time she has left, and clutching at any straw of hope I can.

She sees what I'm doing, and I immediately feel the tension in the air.

'Come on, Mill,' she chides, and her expression makes it clear that saying no isn't an option. I know she hates that I'm doing this. I feel guilty, but, even as I close the lid and get up to follow her, I know I won't stop doing it. I can't.

It's a Saturday, so the house is full of noise and mess and laughter, and if I try, I can pretend that we're a normal happy family; that this spectre doesn't loom over everything now.

But it's okay. The mood lightens as soon as we go into the kitchen.

We're going to make several things today – coconut Bakewells, jam tarts and fairy buns. They're all recipes from Angie's now very dog-eared Be-Ro cookbook – the one her mam gave her just after we got married. She'd sent away for it when it was on offer on bags of Be-Ro flour, back in the seventies – who'd have thought it would still be going so strong?

'Oh, Mill,' Angie laughs, once she's had me put on a pinny. 'You look okay with that on, honest. I wish one of your mates were round to see it!' And, drawn by the sound of her laughter, which they always are, all the kids come in to see what's going on. They've been running around all morning, traipsing back and forth, round and round, in and out of the garden, but the spectacle of their dad in a comedy apron, trying to make buns, proves too much of a show to resist. Soon the youngest five are all crammed into the kitchen with us, Jake – who can't stop giggling – setting off little Corey, while Angie barks orders like a miniature sergeant major. The power's gone to her head now, I can tell.

The children gather round – they all pull chairs up to the kitchen counter, so they can stand on them, all the better to 'help'. All bar Ella, who is perched on Angie's hip, just as she always is. First thing, of course, is to mix up some pastry dough, and, perhaps sensing that it might be a bit complicated for me, she gives me Ella, and does that job herself.

'We always need to make extra pastry,' she tells me, as she mixes it. 'So the kids can make some little tarts as well.'

Jade and Jake are already squabbling over who gets which pastry cutters, while Connor, being the canny one, makes a beeline for the rolling pin, wrestling it from little Corey like a pro. Who'd have thought a piece of dough could create so much excitement?

'There,' Angie says, 'some for you, and some for you . . .'

Somehow the bowl of flour and fat has disappeared – in what felt like moments – and been replaced by a smooth ball of floury dough. How did *that* happen? She gets the rolling pin back off Connor, so she can roll the biggest piece out, turning it on the floured worktop as she goes. Once again, within minutes, the bun tin is lined with little circles, and, though I'm trying to take in her instructions about cutting and re-rolling and not handling it too much, I know that what she's achieved in a matter of a few minutes would, if left to me, take half a day.

'Right,' she says, refusing to help any more now she's got me started, 'here's what you have to do next. You need two ounces of sugar and two ounces of marge. Put it in that bowl there and cream it together.'

I weigh and add the ingredients she passes to me, one by one, then, while she supervises the children's pastry creations, I beat it the way she's shown me – which is fast and pretty furious. And in no time I have a pretty impressive mixture on my hands. Perhaps I will be okay at this after all.

'Done it, sir,' I say proudly, while the children smile and giggle.

'Right,' Angie says, still sounding like someone senior in the army. 'Now you need two ounces of coconut and an egg.'

I add the coconut, and get an egg out of the egg box, but before I add it I stop and look at it. Then at the children, who can sense mischief and have stopped cutting out their tart cases, then at Angie, then back to the egg. She's got her back to me now, standing at the worktop, checking one of the recipes. I look at the kids again, and slowly raise my eyebrows.

'Do it!' Jade cries, clapping her hands. 'Do it, Dad. Get her!'

'Yeah!' the others chorus. 'Do it, Dad! Smash it!'

Hearing them, Angie cottons on and finally lifts her eyes, and, looking up, sees the egg hovering above her head. 'Mill,' she warns, 'I only washed my hair this morning. So just you dare.'

Which is like a red rag to a bull, especially with such an enthusiastic audience. I duly break the egg over the top of her head.

'I'll get you back,' she says, as the yolk snags on her eye-lashes. 'Just you wait, Mill. I'll get you back.'

*

Angie began radiotherapy as soon as she came out of hospital, returning to Sheffield for her treatment twice a week, while I stayed at home to look after the boys. The hospital provided a car for her and, the first time it pulled up outside our house, we noticed there was a young woman already in it. It turned out her name was Jane and she was off for radiotherapy as well and, as she lived nearby, the same car took them both.

Jane lived in Cudworth, about two miles from where we lived, and, understandably, they soon became very close. One day, however, about a month into Angie's treatment, the car turned up as usual, but it was empty, and we wondered if perhaps she was poorly. When Angie returned from treatment that day, however, she immediately burst into tears: Jane had died. And what made it worse was that she'd not long given birth to a baby, just months before finding out her cancer had returned.

This upset Angie dreadfully, as anyone could imagine, and a couple of months later, while we were in Cudworth cemetery putting some flowers on her gran's grave, she decided she'd see if she could find Jane's as well. It took a while, but we found it, among the recently dug graves, so I drove us back to the florist to get some more flowers. Angie cried almost all the way home.

But we had to be positive, because now there was no reason not to be. And, as the weeks passed and we returned to our everyday existence, the spectre of cancer loomed less large in our lives. We had our growing boys, a supportive family, and everything to look forward to. Yes, Angie had lost her breast but she didn't let it get her down. She didn't even want a reconstruction.

She'd been clear on that since the day of her op. 'So what do you think?' she'd asked. It had been only the second day afterwards, the first time we were alone on the ward together, and could take a proper look at the surgeon's handiwork.

'It's not that bad,' I said, and I meant it. I was surprised just how neat it looked.

'You sure, Mill?' she said. 'You sure you don't mind looking at this? And *please* be honest.'

I said what I always did. That I loved her, I fancied her. That it was her and she was perfect. Always had been, always would be. Just as she was. 'But if *you* want a reconstruction,' I told her, 'then you should have it.'

She took another look, then pulled her top back down, decided. 'That's it, then. I'm not. Why would I want to go through another blinking operation when I don't need to? There's only you who's going to see it, Mill, after all.'

So that was that. There was no further talk of reconstruction. Though, as it turned out, I wasn't the last to see it. On the way home from the hospital she wanted to stop at their Neil's and see Diane.

Now it was just a case of taking regular medication: a course of tamoxifen, to be taken for five years. And the consultant made it clear that, though there was *lots* to look forward to, in some cases it mustn't be just yet.

'You mustn't fall pregnant while you're on this medication,' he told her. 'Because it's a powerful drug and could harm an unborn baby. So having another one just yet is a definite no-no.'

His expression seemed to suggest that, with three boys already, it was probably the last thing on our minds in any case. And he was right, as far as I was concerned. We had more than enough on our plates already, what with just getting over the scare of Angie's cancer and with three energetic little kids running around. And, besides, all I cared about was Angie getting well again. Which meant her body needed rest – not to carry another baby. And we were busy: I was still doing long shifts down Pontefract Pit and Angie had a physically demanding part-time job cleaning for the high school behind our house. No, I thought, we're definitely not thinking of having any more children.

But I hadn't reckoned on what was going on inside Angie's head.

'Mill,' she said one night as we cuddled on the sofa, relaxing, and the three boys were finally all asleep in bed, 'do you think, once I've finished taking all this medication, that we could think about having another baby?'

I was shocked – but even more shocked by how immediately I warmed to the idea. But, then again, not so shocked. Wasn't I one of eight myself? And five years was a long time – in five years, little Reece would be seven. It would be fine, I thought. A plan. It *would* be something to look forward to. Yes, it would be a stretch financially, but we'd cope – we weren't big spenders. And, besides that, I'd never deny my wife anything – not anything that it was in my power to give her, anyway. And definitely not when it came to more kids –

she was born to have them. 'Course we can,' I said. 'You know that. You can have anything you want, love.'

'Really?' she said, her face alight with excitement, her eyes huge.

'Really,' I agreed, laughing. 'You can have as many as you like.'

But I never thought she'd actually take me literally.

It's the laughter I think I'll miss more than anything.

The Bakewells and fairy buns and tarts are in the oven now, together with all the pastry creations the kids have made from the scraps, and the whole of the downstairs smells of coconut and strawberry jam and cake. The kitchen's trashed, and, while I set about clearing up, I can not only see them all, out in the garden, but can hear them all as well. The four of them and Angie, all running about – whooping and shouting and giggling as they play chase, while Ella Rose sits in her high chair, sipping juice and watching me wash up. I stand in front of the sink, listening to them all in the garden, and try to imagine life without the sound of Angie's laughter – and I can't.

And, naturally, she does get me back for the egg incident. She times it perfectly. She waits till the afternoon, when the cakes and tarts are out of the oven, and Reece is home from work. The kids are clamouring for them – Reece too, now – and the kitchen's once again spotless, when she ambles in, hair freshly washed, and in her coat.

'Just off to check in on Mam and Dad,' she says, leaning in for a kiss.

But, as she kisses me, she also pulls an egg from her pocket and, before I even realise what she's got and what she's doing, the job is done. With one smooth move on Angie's part, *I'm* now the one who has egg on his face.

'See you later!' she calls, leaving before I can smear her with yolk. I can still see her laughing all the way down the road.

Chapter 5

It's well into May now and, with the days getting longer, we decide to take the younger children away on a week's holiday for the upcoming summer half-term. And, almost as quickly as we've made that decision, we make another – that it'll be to Thornwick Bay.

Thornwick Bay is a very special place to us. It's a sprawling caravan park that sits at the top of Flamborough Head, close to the little seaside town of Bridlington, on the east coast of Yorkshire. And to us it's one of the most beautiful places on earth. I've been going there since I was a four-year-old. It was the first time my mam and dad had ever taken us there on holiday, and we liked it so much we went back every year.

My brother Les – who never married and still lives in my parents' house today, along with Glenn – bought a caravan for the family to use back in the mid-seventies, and I have wonderful memories of it, particularly the year I passed my driving test, when Angie and I would drive up there on weekends to join the rest of the family, both feeling very flash and grown-up in my souped-up Ford Capri. There's not been a year since that we haven't gone and stayed there at some point; some years we'd go two or three times, because Angie loves it there so much, particularly the view from the cliffs.

And a holiday, of course, means doing some holiday shopping. And Angie decides that I need some instruction in the business of buying the children's clothes.

'You need some instruction in shopping, full stop, Mill,' she tells me, as we drive to the local supermarket. We're going to do our big weekly food shop as well today, so we've already done the shopping list, and dropped off Ella with my brother Glenn, who loves having her. He's a couple of years older than I am, but, like Les, he's never married or had kids, and he's the only one of my brothers who's never been a miner.

Glenn's kind-hearted and sensitive, and has a really lovely nature. He's struggled with depression over the years, which is why he's not been able to work much, but despite that – perhaps partly because of it, so patient is he – he has always been the best uncle ever. Being at home, he's always been such a support to me and Angie, always taking the kids for walks down to the park or to help him tend the vegetables in his allotment; and, as he's never been much of a one for going out, he's always been happy to babysit for us, if we wanted a night out for a special occasion.

I turn to Angie, who's sitting there grinning. 'Cheek!' I retort. Because, if there's one thing she's good at, it's going shopping. With Angie never having driven, I've always taken her. And, being the man, I know my place. As with almost every other man I see in Asda, my speciality is pushing the trolley for Angie, always having it at exactly the right place so every time she grabs something off the shelves she can turn right around and put it in.

Which is actually quite an art, as I am quick to point out, as we pull into the supermarket car park. 'And I must have pushed supermarket trolleys for enough miles to go right round the world,' I finish. 'I can push trolleys for Yorkshire – with or without children in them, come to that.'

Angie laughs. She seems happy today, and I know it's because we've booked Thornwick. And I'm glad. Now we have something to look forward to. 'Mill, that's not exactly shopping, is it?' she says, rolling her eyes. 'You've got to plan your meals, work out what you need, know what it's going to come to, remember what you're running out of, look at what's on special offer and think whether you can use it. *That's* shopping.'

And, of course, she's right. When you've as many kids as we have, and are on a very tight budget – which we always are, especially since I stopped working – that's a real mission. And, as I walk behind her into the supermarket, I feel a welling of mild panic, realising just how big a task lies ahead of me.

It will be a *huge* task, and I'd be a fool to think otherwise. I am a man. And we have always run our home traditionally. Which means we both have specific jobs we've always done. I am good on: decorating, gardening, driving elderly relatives to hospitals, running errands, getting prescriptions, digging holes, unblocking drains, lifting heavy children, fixing push-bikes and skateboards, carrying stuff, being strong, knocking together rabbit hutches (not to mention aviaries for housing birds of prey), drilling things – particularly drilling things – and washing up.

But where d'you start with all *this* stuff? It's one thing coming in here just to browse, or to pick up a couple of things, but this is the first time I think I've ever really had to stop and consider what decisions Angie makes before she buys the things she does, and rejects the ones she doesn't.

'Fresh foods,' she's saying to me, as we pass the cream and milk and butter. 'Think before you buy anything that's not going to keep, because if you buy too much you'll just end up throwing stuff away. Try to think of things that keep, or you'll be having to go shopping all the time, too.' She smiles. 'And the novelty will wear off, Mill, trust me. In no time.'

I'm affronted. 'I come every week with you, don't I?' I argue.

Angie gives me an old-fashioned look and a short lecture about the difference between coming food shopping and the business of having to *think* about food all the time – what to eat, what to make, what to buy in order to make it – week after week after week.

And it's not just food, either. It's all the other stuff as well. We're at the laundry aisle now, and I realise I don't know where to start there, either. It seems such a massive and intim-idating explosion of shapes and colours. Why do some people do their washing using little pouches of sparkly liquid, while others heft boxes the size of coffee tables home? What's fabric conditioner *for* exactly? And why, as I remember Angie telling me the other day, must you use it on everything except towels?

My education in this regard is clearly going to be an important one. And it's nowhere as clear as when we head to the clothes section. I have almost no experience of clothes shopping for the children. I've never needed to. Angie goes shopping with her mum every week in Barnsley to do that; it's something they've done for years. It's one of the reasons Angie was so thrilled to have two daughters, so she could go shopping with them just as her mum's always done with her. It's a horrible thought to pop into my mind and I wish it hadn't. Jade's only eight now, and I can't bear to think of all the years ahead of her when she won't have her mum to go shopping with. And little Ella – she's never even going to know what that feels like. It's so unfair.

I watch Angie, just ahead of me, and wonder what she's thinking, as she weaves between the racks of brightly coloured children's summer clothes. Is she thinking the same thing as I am? That this might be the last summer left for her? God, I hope not.

I try to get myself back on track, before she turns around and catches my eye.

She swivels round just then. 'Right,' she says. 'We probably need to grab them all a couple of sets of shorts and T-shirts. Oh, and some new plastic sandals for the beach. How about you take a look in the boys' section and see what you can find for Jake and Corey, while I see what I can find for the girls?' She grins at me. 'That won't be too complicated for you, will it?'

She's right to sound sarcastic. On the odd occasion when I have been put in charge of getting anything for any of the kids single-handed, I haven't exactly made a good job of it. Being logical, I'd always go by the ages on the labels – Angie doesn't need to: she always tells by looking – but I don't think there's been a time when anything I've bought on that basis has ever been the right size, even though it's not as if our kids were all weird shapes.

And I remember the time when I picked out this nice Mickey Mouse T-shirt for Connor for some holiday we were going on. He must have been about four at the time and he loved Mickey Mouse, so I thought it was perfect. But, when I got home and showed Angie, she just burst out laughing. 'Oh, Mill, that's a pyjama top, you nutter!'

I have so much to know about so many things. I just pray there will be long enough to learn it.

Our Jack Russell, Penny, had died just before Angie got ill, so the first thing I did after she began getting better was go out and buy her a new puppy. We all missed Penny. We'd acquired her back in 1985, just a couple of months after we were wed and had moved into our first home in Shafton. Penny lived in Grimethorpe and had a very neglectful owner. Every time we went home to visit either of our parents, we'd be likely to see her roaming the streets.

'You know what we should do?' Angie had said one time when we were over, and Penny had ambled over hoping to be petted. 'We should ask him if he'd let us have her. He clearly doesn't want her, now, does he?'

I wasn't sure. People are apt to get defensive about their animals, however it is they treat them. But Angie was determined. As she said, we had nothing to lose by asking, did we? And, to my surprise, the man was only too happy to agree; he said he just didn't have the time for her any more.

Penny had been a wonderful little dog, and had such a gentle nature, never minding if the boys pulled her around, as boys tend to. I don't think we ever once heard her growl. And, now Angie's ordeal was finally over, it seemed the perfect time to replace her. It would be something new to focus on – a new member of the family, and, as Angie had always said that what she'd most love was a little sausage dog, I went and found her a little dachshund, from a local breeder.

Angie called her Poppy, and she was tiny too. She was only a few weeks old when we got her, and I'm sure the boys wore her out – little Reece, who was a typical two-year-old, in particular. So it was just as well she was another dog with a calm temperament. He would do that typical toddler thing of trying to pick her up all the time. And then, when he'd done that, he'd do that other typical toddler thing, as soon as she wriggled: dropping her again, on her head.

Life felt good again, and we soon settled back into a familiar routine, me grafting down the pit while Angie looked after the boys and ran the home. And somehow the years passed and we got to the spring of 1998, and the magic day of Angie's five-year appointment. She'd been to the hospital a month before to have a scan and some blood tests, and today she had another appointment to see the oncologist to get the results and see about stopping the tamoxifen.

I felt so nervous, sitting there in the cramped, cream-painted office, as tense and agitated as Angie was calm. She got straight to the point, though. So perhaps she wasn't *that* calm.

'So?' she said. I don't think she could bear the suspense a minute longer.

'You're in remission,' said the oncologist, and we both let out sighs of relief, even though I don't think I even realised I'd been holding my breath. He smiled. 'So I'm glad to say that I can now take you off your medication, and there's no reason why you shouldn't live a long and happy life.'

So that was that. It felt a little as if we'd been released from a kind of prison. You don't talk about this stuff, but it was always there, at the back of both our minds.

Angie was grinning from ear to ear, she looked so happy that day. I said so.

'Ah, but y'know what would make me *really* happy,' she giggled, as we crossed the hospital car park and climbed into the car.

'Go on,' I said. 'What would make you *really* happy?'

'To try for another baby,' she said immediately. 'Right away.'

'Whoah!' I said. I was smiling from ear to ear as well now. I must have looked like a proper Cheshire cat. But I shook my head, even so. 'I think we should at least wait till we're home, Ange, don't you? Someone might see us if we try here.'

Angie sighed theatrically. 'Oh, Mill, you are *such* a spoilsport!' Then she laughed that big laugh of hers, and carried on laughing, on and off, all the way home. And it took us a while to get home as well. First we stopped round her brother Neil's so she could tell him the good news, then at her mam and dad's house, and then, finally, to my mam's, where we stayed the obligatory half an hour. That was the rule: you couldn't call at my mam's without stopping for a cuppa. The kettle would be on as soon as you walked through the door, and all the mugs would be down off the shelves ready. I felt as if I was floating as we walked those last few yards back to ours. Angie was okay. It was over. We could get on with our lives now. It was a day I wouldn't forget in a hurry.

And I'd promised her we could try for another baby. So we did try – pretty hard – and, in June 1999, Angie gave birth to our fourth son. We called him Connor. He was a big baby – nine pounds, even though Angie was so tiny – and also robust, which was good, because his three older brothers were all keen to help out in looking after him. And, even though the surgeon had removed Angie's left breast, she still managed to breastfeed him. I was so proud of her.

I thought she might be disappointed to have another boy, but she wasn't. She was in her element with her little quartet of lads to run around after. 'And besides,' she joked, 'it gives me a brilliant excuse, doesn't it? To try for another one!'

So we did try again. And we got two.

Chapter 6

Is packing suitcases for a holiday an art or a science? It's the end of May, and we're off on our holiday, and my next lesson, though not as vexing as trying to knit hair, exposes yet another gaping hole in my knowledge.

However, when it comes to gaping holes, the opposite applies if you're packing suitcases: just how do you fit everything in? And with so many children, little Corey and Ella particularly, there is so much to remember to take. Bedding, for example, which would never have occurred to me. What feel like forty-seven different items of 'essentials' that have never crossed my mind, that have always just 'appeared'. Bite cream and rash cream. Plasters and nail scissors. Colouring books. Seasick pills. Ella's comfort blanket. Connor's coursework for school. Corey's *Toy Story* figures. Jake's Nintendo DS. Jade's roller boots. And to think I thought my feat – fitting everything in the car – was some sort of superior, macho talent.

And, once the packing's finally done, that's the next job. I'm outside the house, standing in the road, the various cases and bags and boxes piled around me. Angie, meanwhile, has popped back inside to change Ella and make sure all the other kids use the toilet before we go.

'Da-*ad*?' asks Connor, in the sort of voice I know well, the sort of voice that means he wants to get round me.

'Con-*nor*,' I reply, trying to shoehorn in all the last bits and bobs. 'Go on, then. What is it you're after?'

He comes round to the side of our hired people carrier and starts to help me, picking up and passing the last few stray carrier bags. 'I was just wondering,' he says. 'Can I bring the laptop?'

He's referring to the old one we passed on to the kids to share. With so many of them, it gets a *lot* of use.

'No, you can't, love.' It's Angie's voice. I didn't even realise she was back out here.

'Oh, but *Mum*,' Connor argues, turning round. 'What about my coursework?'

She narrows her eyes as she begins strapping Ella into her baby seat. 'Why d'you need the laptop to finish your coursework, love?'

Connor pouts. 'Because I might need to look something up for it, mightn't I?'

Angie's eyes narrow further. 'Hmm,' she says. 'This is the first I've heard of any looking-up needing doing. *Writing*-up, yes, but not looking-up, from what I saw. Besides,' she says, 'even if you *do* need to look up something, there'll be plenty of time to do that once we're home.'

I stop what I'm doing. 'You sure, love? If he needs it, there's still some room in here, and—'

'Mill, he *doesn't* need it. Connor, I know full well why you want to take the laptop. It's so you can sit on Facebook or MSN or whatever, chatting to your mates, isn't it?'

Connor's lack of a denial seems to confirm it, and she shakes her head. 'No laptop,' she says firmly, passing me the last of the towels and tea towels. 'This is supposed to be a family holiday. Some time to spend together, doing fun things *together*. We're going to Thornwick Bay to escape the outside world for a bit, okay?' And, though she doesn't so much as even glance in my direction, I know the person she's really talking to is me.

Thornwick Bay is probably one of our favourite places in the world, so it's no surprise that the kids are all a bit hyper and overexcited by the time the loading-up is almost done. And me too. I can't wait to get there, and I know Angie will feel just the same. It's as if, the minute we drive through the entrance and see the sea, all our cares will melt away. It never fails. I'm fast-forwarding in my mind now, to when we're there and can finally relax; to when the kids'll all be playing and we can sit down and have a much-needed cup of tea before we start unpacking the car.

We always try to book the same chalet every time – number ten. It's in a great position because it looks out over the big children's playing field, so we can keep an eye on the little ones while they play. Mind you, I think, before we can *un*pack, we have to finish packing, and now half a dozen new things have suddenly appeared, I realise that'll be a job and a half. It sometimes seems that the amount of stuff they all expect me to fit in gets more and more every time we go. It's going to be a struggle, even with the roomy people carrier, and I make a mental note that we need to find a way to be able to afford to buy something bigger than our own car, such as the old Shogun we used to have before its engine blew up. Since then, I've given up on owning an expensive seven seater. Just got a reliable regular car and hired people movers on the odd occasion they're necessary.

Except thinking about car options feels a thought too far, because it just reminds me of the future, which is a bad place. I need to fix firmly on the here and now.

'You know what?' I tell Angie, smiling as an act of will to try to shake the thought away. I'm trying to make space for Jade's doll's pram, which is tricky. 'I don't know why I didn't just hire a lorry and be done with it!'

'Now that's a thought,' Angie agrees. 'I've always fancied myself sitting way up in a big artic. We could do CB radio, and have one of those little beds up behind the cab.'

'An' a mini TV,' chimes in Connor, who's now passing me his skateboard. 'I've seen that on the telly. They make them like proper little rooms.'

But no laptops, I think. Not for us. Angie's right. This is supposed to be about escaping. I get the skateboard in, and allow myself a moment of pride in my achievement. There might be lots I can't do, but at least I can do this. Though as I manage to squeeze in the very last item – Jake's precious scooter – I find myself ambushed by another horrible thought: of all the extra space there'll be available when neither Angie nor her things are going to be here.

Pushing thoughts like this aside is becoming increasingly

hard to do. *Stop it*, I tell myself, as I watch her now settling the kids into their booster seats. We have lots of time together still. Angie is well just now. There are still chemotherapy options open to us. Live in the moment.

Trouble is, I think as I head back up the path to lock the house, that the moments are going so fast.

Angie was in fits, that day, telling me about how we were expecting twins. It was in the spring of 2002 that we found out she was pregnant, and, once again, she was really excited at the thought of having a new baby in the house. By now, Ryan and Damon were in high school, Reece just finishing his time at primary, and little Connor would soon be going on three.

Life was busy. I was still working at Pontefract Colliery as a tunneller, and was on a complicated rota of eight- and twelve-hour shifts. Nights were the worst, because I'd set off at 5 p.m. to start my shift at six, then work through till 6 a.m., getting home around seven, just as the rest of the family were getting up.

I didn't go to bed then: I'd stay up to take the older boys to school for Angie, so it would save her doing the walk with little Connor. Then I'd get my head down, for perhaps three hours or so – four, if I was lucky – then have a bit of lunch with them before Angie went to work. I'd take Connor then, to go and pick the boys up from school again, then, before I knew it, Glenn was round – he minded the kids till Angie was home again – and I was back off to work to do my next shift!

It was all a bit of a military exercise, as it is for so many families. And, looking back, I realise it was a pretty complicated way to live a life. But with the kind help of our families – my brother Glenn in particular – we managed, just as everyone else did.

Today was a good day, though. A relatively normal day shift. And I'd been able to finish a little early, as well, since it was a pretty waterlogged tunnel we'd been working in. And better still, right away, as I opened the back door, I could smell curry. A pretty good day so far all round, then. And one that was about to get better. Angie was in the kitchen, Connor playing on the floor beside her, and when she turned to greet me she was grinning from ear to ear.

'What?' I said enquiringly. But, as soon as she'd start telling me, she'd just burst out laughing and have to stop again.

'*What*, love?' I said, mystified. 'Go on – what's so funny?'

'Oh, Mill,' she said, once more composing herself. 'You are *never* going to believe this. I can hardly believe it myself.'

'Believe what?' I said, not knowing what she was on about at that point. I'd been gone since 5 a.m., before she was up, and I'd completely forgotten about today's hospital appointment. It was only when she went to get something from her handbag that it clicked that she'd been there that morning. But I still couldn't work out why she was so excited.

'Sit down,' she commanded. She had something in her hand now.

'Sit down? Why?' I glanced towards the cooker. 'Dinner's not ready yet, is it?'

She pulled out a chair for me. 'Yes, sit down, Mill. You're going to need to when you see this!'

She handed me the piece of paper now, and now I had it in my hand I could immediately see it was the scan photo. Not that it looked any different from the others, as far as I could tell.

'Surprise!' she said, pointing out the two tiny hearts, then bursting into huge peals of laughter.

I gaped, realising what I was seeing. I looked again, then, to double-check, as I couldn't quite believe it. She was pulling my leg, surely? She was always one for joking like that.

'It's never,' I said.

'Mill, it *is*,' she said. 'It's twins, honest! Isn't that exciting? Oh, Mill, can you imagine it?' She did a little mime. 'Imagine holding two in your arms at once? Oh, and I can dress 'em the same – if they're both the same sex, that is, obviously, and—'

'Hold up,' I said. 'I'm still trying to get my head round this. *Twins?*'

'Oh, it's not that surprising, when you think about it, Mill. Look at our Linda. She's got twins, hasn't she?' Linda was Angie's cousin, and she was right. She did have them. Wow, I thought, taking it in. We were actually going to have twins.

And, as it sank in, I realised it was a really good feeling. I stretched my arms up above my head, easing the knots in my back out. 'Hey, Angie,' I said. 'I reckon I must be getting better with age, then. I can knock 'em out two at a time now!'

Angie laughed as she picked up Connor. 'Listen to him,' she said. 'Thinks he's some kind of superstud now! And less of the you, Mill, if you don't mind – I think you'll find it'll be *me* knocking them out.'

But, if we were excited then, it was as nothing compared with how happy we'd be at Angie's next scan. It was at twenty weeks, just after Connor's third birthday, and on this occasion, because of the shifts I was doing that week, I was able to take her myself.

Angie was fizzing like a bottle of pop all the way to the hospital and had hopped up on the bed beside the ultrasound machine before the operator had hardly closed the door.

'This is it, Mill,' she said, grabbing hold of my hand as I sat down on the chair beside the bed. 'We're going to know. Oh, I'm that excited, I really am!' She turned to the operator, who was busy pouring squiggles of gel on her tummy. 'We want to know the sex,' Angie said. 'Did I tell you that? We definitely want to know. We've got four boys, you see, so we're hoping we might be in with the chance of a girl now. What with there being two of them.'

The ultrasound operator smiled. She was a lovely young woman with dark hair and a wide smile. 'Well,' she said, sitting down at the machine, 'let's see if we can get one for you, shall we?' She grinned. 'I've got three girls myself, and they're a handful.' She turned to me, then. 'I bet you'd love a little girl as well, wouldn't you? And spoil her rotten, I'll bet. Dads always do.'

She was spot on. As the only girl in a family of eight, my sister definitely was spoilt.

'So, let's see, then, shall we?' the operator said. 'Here we go.' And as she swept the paddle across Angie's tummy we watched the pictures form and change. 'Ah,' she said, finally, pressing a button to freeze the screen. Then she pointed. 'So . . . this one is definitely a boy,' she told us. 'Let's see if it's his twin sister down here.'

She pressed the button a second time and, as the picture started changing, I felt Angie's grip on my hand tighten slightly. I knew it wouldn't be the end of the world if she wasn't carrying a daughter. Having a little girl would be the icing on the cake for us both, obviously, but, if it turned out she was carrying boys again, then so be it. I knew she would love them with all her heart. But I also knew how much she wanted to have a daughter too, so I crossed the fingers of my free hand, even so.

'Ah,' said the operator again. 'And here . . . yes, I *think* so.' She turned the paddle this way and that so she could get a clearer view. Then she grinned at us. 'It looks like you got your wish,' she said, 'because this one is *definitely* a girl.'

Angie burst into tears as soon as she heard that, she was so happy. 'Oh, a girl, Mill!' she sobbed. 'We've finally got our girl! I can't wait to get home and tell Mum!'

So she did, just as soon as we were back from the hospital, and she talked of nothing else for the rest of the night. All the things they'd do, all the things she'd teach her, all the beautiful clothes she'd dress her in.

'And it's not just me, Mill,' she said that night, once we'd put the boys to bed. 'Just think – it's happened. You're going to have a daughter. And one day you're going to be walking her up the aisle.'

It was an exciting time. And also a busy one. Within a matter of weeks we'd be a family with six kids to run around after, so we had quite a lot of organising to do. Once again the drawers started filling up with new baby clothes – but this time round, because we already had enough boys' things to open a shop with, almost all the things Angie brought home from her shopping trips with her mum were frilly and girly and pink.

Jake and Jade were born on a chilly November day in 2002, and I don't think, as a family, we'd ever been happier. Yes, things were tighter than they'd ever been, but we didn't want to spend money going out, anyway. Angie was never happier than when we were all together on a Saturday night, with a takeaway Chinese, the kids all in pyjamas, and she, with a baby in each arm – she even managed to breastfeed – glued to her beloved *Pop Idol* or *The X Factor*. And I was just happy that she was happy. Why wouldn't I have been? We had everything we needed right at home.

But can you be *too* happy? Was fate out to test us? I have no idea, but we were about to find out.

Chapter 7

It was one in the morning, in March 2004, and I had a 6 a.m. shift looming. Not the best time to find yourself suddenly awake. But that was what I was: wide awake, all of a sudden. And feeling odd in a way I couldn't put my finger on. I lay still, listening to Angie breathing softly beside me. Other than that the house was silent, and also dark. My only company was the glow of the digital display of my alarm clock, which was set to go off at 4.30.

I was normally a good sleeper, despite my irregular shift patterns – a head-on-pillow, out-like-a-light kind of guy. But for some reason tonight I just couldn't seem to settle again. I tried to work out what had woken me. Was something worrying me subconsciously? It was just so strange to be feeling as I did. It was only after a night shift that I had any trouble sleeping: it's never easy to fall asleep when the rest of the world's awake. But that wasn't the case and I had no idea why I should feel so restless.

It was when I turned over, for the umpteenth time, just to try to get comfortable, that I felt this sharp agonising pain seem to explode in my head. It was a pain the like of which

I'd never felt before, ever. As if someone had punched me in the forehead with the palm of their hand. I'd had headaches before – several recently. But I'd thought they'd been migraines. And they'd been pretty bad, but nothing like this.

Frightened now, I tried to struggle up into a sitting position, but that only made the pain sear through my head even more. Then, without warning, I felt a welling of intense nausea. I knew I was going to be sick and, as I struggled to get out of bed, I couldn't hold it. I lurched forward and vomited all over the bedroom floor.

I tried to swing my legs around properly, conscious of Angie beginning to stir beside me. She was a light sleeper anyway, as mothers so often are, and within seconds she was wriggling up to find out what was wrong. 'Mill?' she said, throwing her covers off. 'What's happened?' But I couldn't manage to form an answer. I was losing focus now, dizzy and disoriented in the darkness. The pain was so intense I couldn't seem to think beyond it. I needed to move – yes, that was it. I needed to get to the bathroom. But when I tried to stand my legs just buckled beneath me.

Angie was up on her feet now, running around the bed to yank the bedroom door open more fully. The smell of the sick was making me want to retch again. 'Ryan!' she was shouting, as light spilt in from the landing. 'Ryan! Wake up! Come and help me!'

I was only dimly aware now of the commotion around me: of Ryan thundering in; of Angie telling him to stay with me; of her rattling down the stairs to call an ambulance.

Then the sensation of being jerked around, as they both struggled to put some clothes on me. I could no longer seem even to move of my own accord now. The pain was overwhelming. What the hell was happening to me? I was terrified.

I remember nothing of the journey to Barnsley District Hospital. The first thing I recall was seeing bright lights above me, and a new smell, a clinical smell, that prickled in my nostrils.

There was someone speaking too. A doctor.

'Mr Millthorpe?' he was saying. 'Can you hear me? We've done a scan, and you've had a brain haemorrhage, so we're going to transfer you to the Sheffield Hallamshire Hospital. Okay?'

I tried to nod, but couldn't. Everything seemed to swim in front of me. The only thing I could hear clearly was the sound of Angie crying.

The next time I woke up I was in a different place, travelling on a trolley. I knew I was moving because there were fluorescent strip lights above me, flashing past. Once again, Angie was beside me, and I could hear her sobbing. She was holding my hand, striding along beside me, the tears streaming down her face. There were several people with us – I saw my brother Malc and my sister-in-law Eileen. And another doctor, who began speaking to me in low and urgent tones. We'd come to a stop now, and there was activity going on all around me.

'Mr Millthorpe,' he was saying. He was wearing scrubs: a

surgeon. 'We're going to have to operate on you. If we don't then it's likely that you'll be dead in twelve hours.'

I couldn't quite take in what he was telling me. I felt Angie squeeze my hand.

'So,' he asked, 'do you feel able to sign the consent form?'

I nodded. What else was I to do? But first, he explained, he needed to make me aware of the risks. And he was frank. 'There's around a thirty per cent chance you will recover fully,' he told me slowly. 'But also a thirty per cent chance you won't survive surgery. Finally, there is a similar chance that you *will* survive the operation – but will also be left brain-damaged.' He paused to let that sink in. 'Do you understand?'

Maths isn't my strong point, but the sums weren't that difficult. I either would die or I might die or I might end up a vegetable. On the other hand, I might be okay. And we had had our share of bad luck. I remember being reassured, thinking that, as if it were yesterday. We had *definitely* had our share of bad luck. 'Don't worry,' I said to Angie, who was standing there, sobbing her heart out. 'I'll be okay, I know I will.'

I took the pen and signed the form then, my hand weak and shaky, and once that was done Angie kissed my cheek and they wheeled me into the operating theatre. I could still hear her crying as the doors closed.

Once I was inside, there was another rush of activity. I could see the surgeon and his assistants attaching cables and tubes to me, and the anaesthetist – a woman – came and stood close beside me. 'Right, Ian,' she told me, pushing a syringe of clear liquid into the cannula they'd fixed in my hand. 'I'm going to put you to sleep now, okay?'

And I remember looking around, taking everything in, and wondering if I'd ever see Angie and the kids again, or whether this brightly lit room, with all its beeping machinery and flashing lights, would be the last thing I'd ever see. The odds definitely weren't in my favour.

There is no celestial score sheet. That much is clear. But when I woke from the operation I felt the luckiest man alive, because it seemed the odds *had* worked in my favour: the first thing I saw was Angie. I was awake. I was alive. She was sitting on a chair close beside me, and so were Malc and Eileen.

'You're going to be okay, Mill,' was the first thing she said to me. 'Everything went fine.'

She leant across then, and kissed me, and smiled that beautiful smile of hers. 'Thank God,' she said quietly. 'I thought I'd lost you.'

I tried to focus on her, but I could see out of only one eye. But her words all made sense to me. I could see her. I had *survived*.

'You're in intensive care,' she explained, as I took in my new surroundings. The strange bed, the many monitors, the tubes that seemed to be attached to every part of me. The smiling male nurse who Angie told me was looking after me.

'My eye ...' I said. 'It's—'

Angie placed a hand over mine. 'It's just the swelling,' she explained to me. 'From the surgery. You're eye's fine.'

And it seemed I *was* fine. I could make sense of things, understand everything Angie was saying to me. Which meant that, so far at least, my brain seemed to be working okay, even if my face felt as big and stretched as a pumpkin.

My brother Barry was there too, I realised, sitting just the other side of me. And it was daytime. Afternoon. Two o'clock, the clock said. And there was my brother, and he was grinning at me. Not crying, but grinning. He pointed towards my head, which he could see and I obviously couldn't, where, unbeknown to me, there was a line of staples that ran from the top of my head right down to just behind my ear.

'I see they've fitted a zip on that head, mate,' he chuckled. 'Tha looks like summat off of *Star Wars*, tha does, young 'un!'

The day after the op I felt well – amazingly well, in fact – and was finally allowed to eat breakfast: a plate of sausage, eggs and beans. I tucked in – I was ravenous – but something was wrong. For some reason, I couldn't seem to taste it. Great, I remember thinking. I've picked up the flu on top of every-thing. Because it wasn't just that: there was also this feeling my nose was blocked, and, whenever I tried to blow it, there was blood.

I didn't think that much about it though – I had more important things to think about. Like getting well again and going home. But it came up again that evening, when Angie and Malc were visiting, and my dinner arrived – beef stew and dumplings.

'That looks nice, that does,' Angie said.

'Yeah, it does,' I agreed, sniffing it. 'I just wish I could taste it. Just my luck to go through brain surgery and then get a bug, eh?'

Again, I didn't dwell on it – I had a bug. I couldn't smell stuff. It was only when I was in the shower a couple of mornings later that it hit me that perhaps there was more going on than just that. Angie had brought in all my stuff for me, including my aftershave – Joop, her favourite – and, when I splashed some on after drying off and, once again, could smell nothing, I actually poured some into my hands. I cupped them and brought them up to my face, really close. But it was the same as with the food. I could smell nothing. Not a thing. Which was weird. Even with a cold, I should be able to smell something as strong as this, shouldn't I? Something had definitely happened with my nose.

I decided to ask the consultant when he came to see me on his ward round later that morning.

'Ah,' he said straightaway. 'That's because of the surgery, I'm afraid.'

He went on to explain that, because the bleed was at the base of my brain, they'd had to physically lift it up to be able to get at and clip the aneurysm, which meant the nerves to my nose had to be severed.

'Will I get my sense of smell back again?' I asked.

'I'm afraid not,' he said. 'Those nerves can't grow back.'

So that was that. And it took a good while to sink in. I would have to live the rest of my life without a sense of smell.

Angie was predictably upbeat about it, however. When she came to see me that night, and I was trying to put on a brave face and mostly failing, she was adamant I look on the bright side. I was alive when there'd been a good chance I'd not make it through. I was still here to see my kids all grow up.

'And there's a thought, Mill,' she said, smiling from ear to ear. 'Just think how much easier you'll find nappy-changing now!'

Angie was right, of course. I should just be grateful to be alive. But I had to spend a full month in hospital, which felt like a lifetime. Angie had been advised that it would be better if the children weren't brought onto the ward, so it was a lonely time. Despite the daily visits from Angie and the rest of the family, the hours stretched interminably, the days seeming endless. I was confined to bed, too, so there was nothing to break the monotony, either. The only excitement to be had was when I was out of bed too long, and got a proper ticking off from one of the nurses.

When the time approached for my discharge, I was counting the days, ticking them off in my head like a prisoner in a cell. I couldn't wait to get home, and was determined that nothing was going to stop that happening. So when, a couple of days before that, I became aware of a pain in my hip when I walked, I said nothing. It would probably *be* nothing, in any case. I was used to keeping fit, so in all probability this was just a niggle from my having been forced to spend so much time in bed. But, almost as soon as I was home, I knew it might be something more serious. As the day had gone on so the pain had been spreading, so much so that, when it got to bedtime, I could hardly move for it.

'Are you coming up?' Angie wanted to know, when she was done with watching telly.

I shook my head. At that moment I couldn't even imagine

getting off the sofa. 'I'll sleep down here, I think,' I told her. 'Go on. You go on up. I'll only keep you awake, tossing and turning.'

'Why?' she wanted to know. 'Are you okay, Mill?'

'I'm fine,' I said, brushing it off. 'Just stiff, that's all. Uncomfortable.'

'Then I'll sleep down here with you.'

'No need,' I said. 'Go on. Go up to bed. You get some sleep.'

I got none. I spent the whole night in terrible pain. By now I could no longer move any part of my body without being in so much agony it made me cry out. What was happening to me to cause this? Was I having another brain haemorrhage? Once again I was terrified and, when Angie came down to see if I was okay, I could keep up the pretence no longer.

'I'm in agony,' I confessed to Angie. 'Every part of my body hurts.'

Angie wasted no time discussing things. She went straight to the phone to call an ambulance. And, with Glenn whistled up to help Ryan mind the little ones, the pair of us headed straight back to the hospital.

Angie came in the ambulance with me, Malc and Eileen following in their car, and by the time we got there my brother Barry had arrived, too. I just couldn't believe quite how terrible I was feeling. I honestly thought I was going to die. How could you feel this bad – and I was feeling worse by the minute – and not have something life-threatening wrong with you?

And it turned out I was right. I did have something life-threatening. They did a lumbar puncture and within the hour they had reached a diagnosis. I had potentially fatal post-operative meningitis and would need to be returned to the Royal Hallamshire. So by ten that night, and with a cock-tail of drugs now being administered intravenously, I was back in the very hospital I'd left the previous morning.

I remember a nurse from that night. I remember asking her right out if I was going to die. And I also remember her frightening reply: 'We're doing everything possible.'

They wanted me to stay in hospital for another three weeks – that was the way it worked: I was hooked up to a drip for an hour or so three times a day, while the antibiotics were given to me intravenously – and that was what I should have done. Having another brush with death, especially so soon after the last one, should have been a signal for me to rest in hospital for as long as it took. But I couldn't bear it. I'd hardly seen my kids for over a month now, and all I wanted was to be home again and feel normal.

And I was glad I badgered the staff into letting me have my drugs at home from a district nurse, because no sooner was I home than we had another trauma. I was sitting indoors wait-ing for the nurse to arrive one day when Angie looked out and saw our little dachshund Poppy lying on the drive, sur-rounded by a pool of blood. 'Quick, Mill,' she said, rushing back in. 'Come outside. Poppy's bleeding.' So I went outside to find Poppy bleeding from her back end, and clearly very ill.

Angie couldn't drive, and I wasn't allowed out yet, so, while Angie rushed in to get a blanket to wrap Poppy up in,

I phoned my brother Malc to see if he could take her to the vet for us. Which he and Terry did, while the nurses came to give me my medication, and it was just after they left that Malc phoned me to say the vet had done an X-ray and that, because Poppy had cancer, it would be kindest just to put her to sleep.

Angie was devastated. She loved Poppy just as much as if she'd been one of her children. I'll never forget the look on her face as she watched Malc get out of the passenger door of Terry's car with Poppy's tiny collar in his hand.

Getting home was good, but, as the weeks passed and I slowly recovered, I began to realise just how much I had lost. It wasn't just my sense of smell I'd have to do without. It seemed I'd also have to do without my work. And not just because of the brain haemorrhage, either. Straight after my operation the consultant had told me that it had been touch and go because of the terrible state my lungs were in. It turned out that the anaesthetist had doubted I'd survive the operation, not just from the haemorrhage, but because my lungs were so weak. Over the years, it seemed mining had quietly taken its toll on me: I had lost 50 per cent of my lung function to chronic obstructive pulmonary disease.

The outlook was suddenly bleak. It would be a year before I'd have a hope of being pronounced fit to return to work, anyway. There was no question I could go back till my symptoms had gone away: as a consequence of the brain haemorrhage I was still suffering regular blinding headaches and blackouts, something that went on for many months.

And, though I still held out hope as the time passed, I think I knew the truth. With the condition of my lungs, I would never pass the medical, even if I made a full recovery from the bleed.

There was no choice for me. My career as a miner was over. I had to take early retirement, aged just forty-two.

It was a very hard transition. I had always loved my job. It was my whole life; it defined me. Yes, it was hard, but it was also a great atmosphere underground. We were a team, and a strong team, who looked out for each other. And there was no finer feeling than coming home from a long shift, and feeling able to relax, knowing I'd done a day's graft, and was providing for my wife and my family.

But I did adjust; I had to. My health mattered to all of us. And I didn't want to end up the way my dad had because of mining, fighting for every breath he took, and taken from life much too early. I was also aware that Angie's family lived to good ages and kept well. What use would I be to her once the kids had grown up if I was half crippled by all the coal dust I inhaled?

It was a shock to us financially. Even with my pension, with six mouths to feed we were poorer than we'd ever been. But, once I got my health back, what I mostly remember about that period was the feeling of actually *being* one of the family. I'd missed out on so much of the children's growing and changing, because I'd always spent so many hours underground. So I relished being there. Perhaps that's what happens when you have such a close brush with your own death: in every sense that matters, life feels so much richer.

In fact, we must have been very happy during that time, looking back. Because Corey Ian came along in 2005. And then, to our delight, we became grandparents as well, Damon and his girlfriend Natalie having a baby boy, Warren, the following year.

Angie was so thrilled – being a grandmother was the best feeling in the world, she said – but it turned out she wasn't quite done with having babies herself. However, when in 2007 she gave birth to our second daughter, Ella Rose, I did joke that perhaps I should find the surgeon who clipped my aneurysm, and see if he'd clip something else for me instead . . .

Chapter 8

Perhaps because everything has changed so radically since she was born, it feels incredible that Ella's soon going to be three and that Ryan has already turned twenty-six. Incredible that Angie's been a mum for more than half her lifetime, and brought eight beautiful children into the world.

And she's done a brilliant job, so she's right to be proud of every one of them. The three oldest boys are all working now, though not following me down the mines. What little was left of the mining industry after the terrible situation in 1984 is only limping along these days – there's no career for them there. But they're still down at the local colliery, in a manner of speaking, working for a firm that operates on the land it used to sit on, building kitchen units – working hard for a good honest wage.

The younger ones are also thriving: Connor's just finishing up in primary school, with Jade and Jake not far behind him. So it's just little Corey and Ella left at home now, and every single second's so precious.

And so heartbreaking to know Angie's going to be taken from us, and that her youngest children are going to have to grow up without their mum. And, with every birthday celebrated, that reality creeps ever closer, however much each is to be a cause for celebration – that she's still here. That she hasn't left us yet.

We're in Toys R Us today, having dropped Ella with Damon's girlfriend, Natalie. Which means she can play with our little grandson Warren for the morning – they are great friends now – while we go and buy her something for her birthday.

It's a place I've been often, but today it feels so different. Because, as soon as we get in there, I begin to see the world through Angie's eyes. Or at least what I assume is the world through Angie's eyes, one in which every little detail must be skewed by the knowledge of how little of it she has left to see.

The age of three is a milestone in a toyshop – a major hurdle. Three equals entry into a whole new realm of playthings, playthings that don't bear the familiar marking: the 'no entry'-style flash across the symbols '0–3'. As we walk I see acres of brightly coloured shelf space, all crammed almost to the rafters with playthings that Angie will never get the pleasure of buying for her children as they grow.

I try to direct my thoughts elsewhere, to do as I'm told and enjoy the moment. And, as I watch Angie cooing indecisively over dolls' clothes and buggies, it occurs to me that, actually, I *am* enjoying the moment. Were it not for death looming, I might not even *be* here, sharing something that Angie clearly loves so much.

But then, at the till, with Ella's presents chosen, she has a rethink.

'Oh, Mill!' she cries, seeing a little white toy dog. It looks like a West Highland terrier, and has a lead attached, so you can pull it, and, to Angie's delight, it even barks as it walks.

'Oh, I don't know which to choose now!' she says, picking up the little dog and cooing over it as if it were real. Angie loves dogs. 'She'd adore this,' she says. 'She could take it out for walks with me and Pebbles, couldn't she?'

We can't afford it, but I tell her to get the dog as well.

I got Pebbles for Angie for Christmas 2006, as a surprise.

We already had Jess by now, but Jess was really Reece's dog. We'd let him have her a few months after we lost Poppy, when Malc's son's dog had puppies and we went round to see them, and Reece fell in love with her on sight. But I knew Angie would really love to have another dachshund, so I searched for a breeder and finally settled on a miniature, red, long-haired bitch, and on Christmas Eve afternoon I told Angie I had some last-minute shopping to do, then drove thirty miles to collect her. I couldn't wait to see Angie's face when I brought her home – well, after her 'where have you been?' face had gone, that is.

Only Reece was in on the plan, so I had to be crafty. I obviously couldn't wrap up an eight-week-old puppy and put her under the tree, so, just before I walked back into the house, I took the tiny trembling scrap of fur from the box she'd travelled home in, undid my jacket zip, and slipped her inside.

Angie was in the living room with the kids, warming her hands by the fire.

'Ay up,' I said, having to do my best not to burst out laughing. 'I've got your Christmas present under my coat, love.'

Angie gave me an old-fashioned look when I said that, but it changed to one of disbelief as I slowly unzipped the jacket and the tiny puppy face suddenly popped out. She was already blooming – she was three months gone with Ella at the time – but now her face lit up brighter than the lights on our Christmas tree. It was such a happy time for us, that year.

But our period of happiness wasn't to last. Angie had this strange cough start up in November 2007, just six months after Ella was born. She just couldn't shake it off and I kept nagging her to see the doctor, but she was her usual robust self and was having none of it.

'I'm *fine*, Mill,' she kept saying to me. 'Stop worrying.'

But I couldn't stop worrying. Suppose it was something serious. I had no reason to think that, because Angie had never smoked, and her breast cancer had been so long ago now that it didn't even register, but, after I'd nearly lost my own life, I was just so conscious that we mustn't ignore things like that. I remembered so well how much it had been on my mind that I might not live to see my children grow up. It was something we'd talked about ever since we'd been teenagers: how hard it would be to live life on our own and how we both wished we'd die before each other.

So I kept nagging, and, when she started getting breathless as well, I made the appointment for her with the GP myself. And drove her there. And went in with her as well.

And the doctor didn't seem to take her cough lightly,

either. He made us an appointment at the hospital for Angie to go and have an X-ray, which came through only a couple of weeks later. And once again I drove Angie and went in too.

'It'll be fine, Mill,' Angie told me as we waited to see the doctor. And then again, once he'd examined her and listened to her chest, and sent us down so she could have her X-ray. 'It won't be anything serious,' she reassured me once she'd come out of the radiology department. 'You'll see. You worry too much, Mill.'

The X-ray done, we went back to the place we'd first waited, and handed over the brown envelope to the receptionist. We were then shown to a cubicle and asked to wait for the doctor, who she told us would come down to see us as soon as he'd looked at the film.

'Mill, I'm gagging,' Angie said, once we'd gone in and sat down. 'My mouth's dry as anything. Go to the hospital shop, will you, and get me some chewing gum and a bottle of pop? We could be here a while, after all, couldn't we?'

I duly went. I was glad to have something to do, because I hated all this waiting, particularly the kind of waiting you had to do when you were in a hospital and the wait was for medical news. I'd done more than my share of that kind of thing for one lifetime. But I mustn't jump the gun. I must keep positive, just as Angie kept telling me. So, as I walked, I tried to talk myself out of this sense of impending doom. Perhaps it would be nothing. Perhaps something not that serious, something treatable. By the time I got the drink and gum and was on my return journey, I think I had almost convinced myself, too. But, when I pulled back the curtain, the doctor was already in the cubicle with Angie, and I could see straightaway from the expressions on both their faces that I was about to hear something really bad.

Angie wasted no time in putting me straight, either. 'It's not good news,' she said, her voice small. 'There's a shadow on my lung.'

She turned back to the doctor, while I just stood there, terrified and gobsmacked, pop in one hand, packet of chewing gum in the other. 'Is it pneumonia?' she asked him. I could hear the anxiety in her voice now.

The doctor shook his head. 'I don't know,' he said. 'And I won't know till we've sent you for a biopsy, I'm afraid.'

I looked at Angie, but she was just nodding calmly at the doctor. 'How soon will it be?' she asked.

'About a week,' the doctor told her. 'Shouldn't be any longer.'

'Around Christmas, then?'

'Yes,' he said. 'Around Christmas.'

Which meant Christmas was difficult, but we still tried to keep our spirits up. After all, we reasoned, the odds were overwhelmingly in Angie's favour. She had never smoked in her life, so what were the chances of it being lung cancer? Very small. And as for her breast cancer – well, it couldn't be anything to do with that, could it? She'd been given the all-clear seventeen years back, so that was history. Pneumonia, we decided. It would most likely be pneumonia, which we knew could be cured. We knew because Angie's sister, another Diane, had had it only the year before. She'd been treated in hospital and now she was as right as rain.

Our appointment to discuss the results of Angie's biopsy came through for a day in early January, just after the kids were back in school. It was dry, but bitterly cold, the frost lingering on the grass and pavements, and, try as I might to keep feeling positive for Angie, fear was creeping around me as surely as the condensation that swirled in the air every time we breathed out. It kept sneaking up on me and ambushing me. What if it *was* something serious? What then? As we sat in the waiting room I gripped Angie's hand so tightly that I nearly cut off her circulation. I didn't know what else to do. She, meanwhile, just sat there, staring into space. Please God, I thought. *Please* let it be good news.

'Angela Millthorpe!'

We both jumped when we heard Angie's name being shouted, and I felt this tingle of fear shoot down my spine. This was it. We stood up and followed the nurse into the consulting room and took the two seats beside the doctor's desk.

He was looking at his computer monitor, but then he looked at Angie.

'This shadow on your lung,' he said to her quietly. 'Do you have any ideas what it might be?'

Angie looked confused that he should ask her. 'Is it pneumonia?' she asked him.

He shook his head. 'No, it's not that. Do you have any other ideas as to what it could be?'

Angie thought for a while. 'Well,' she said eventually, 'I did have breast cancer way back in 1993 ...'

She trailed off. I think we both knew from the doctor's face what was coming.

'I'm so sorry,' he said slowly. 'But it *is* your breast cancer.' He paused, then. 'It's returned and has spread to your lung.'

I just sat there, dazed with shock. I couldn't believe it. Her *breast* cancer? It seemed inexplicable. After seventeen years, and five more children, that tiny lump in Angie's breast – a lump that had been no bigger than a pea – had returned and was about to tear our world apart. I tried to hold back the tears but it was an impossible task. I could hardly bear to look at Angie for fear of breaking down completely, but, when I did, I could see that she was shaking. Shaking, but not crying. She was holding herself together. It was *she* who put her arms around *me*.

'Come on, Mill,' she said, squeezing me. 'I'm okay. You'll be okay.'

But how could she be when her cancer had come back? How could I be okay? How could either of us?

'I'm going to refer you to see an oncologist,' the doctor told us, as we sat there clinging to one another. 'To discuss your options. As soon as possible, obviously.'

I could barely take anything in after that. There was a nurse in the room as well, and now she came across and placed a hand on Angie's shoulder. 'Would you like to go to a private room?' she asked gently. 'To be on your own for a while?'

Angie shook her head. 'No,' she said. 'Come on, Mill, take me home. I just want to go home, please.'

The nurse nodded. And, as she led us out of the doctor's

office, I remember all the people in the waiting room, seeing the expressions on all their faces, and how I could tell they knew we'd had the worst news ever just by the state of us. As if we both had the word 'cancer' written on our foreheads.

By the time we got to the car, however, we were both determined to try to be positive. We mustn't think the worst before we knew the full facts, after all. Yes, the cancer had come back but that didn't mean we shouldn't be hopeful. 'Let's at least wait till we've seen the oncologist,' Angie was saying. 'Who knows? They might be able to remove the tumour like they did last time, mightn't they? And then give me chemo. It might be all right. It worked last time, didn't it?'

I agreed that it did. I wiped my eyes on the tissue the nurse had given me, and when we got in the car I leant across and kissed Angie's wet cheek. 'Yes, love,' I said firmly. 'Maybe that's what they'll do.'

The two-week wait to see the oncologist felt interminable. Now we knew the cause of Angie's symptoms, every minute felt like forever – a forever in which the cancer in her lung could grow unchecked. And the more it grew, the harder it would be to get rid of it.

But we were soon to be disabused of any hope of their getting rid of it, anyway – within minutes of sitting down with the doctor.

'I'm so sorry,' he said gently to Angie, 'but this time I'm afraid we can't cure you, Mrs Millthorpe. All we can do is try to prolong your life with chemotherapy.'

We were both stunned. I could tell Angie was numb with shock, hearing that. Her whole body was rigid, her skin pale, her mouth set. This was the worst news ever. *They couldn't cure her. They could only try to prolong her life.* But for how long? I wanted to scream, shout, punch something, *anything* – it felt so unfair. So brutal. So final. It was like hearing that an innocent woman had just been given the death penalty without reprieve. I really *was* going to lose her now. We all were. This was it.

We both of us cried, for the whole journey home. Angie was sobbing, really sobbing, her shoulders heaving in spasms as the tears dripped onto her lap. I could hardly drive the car. I couldn't see for looking. The thought of living without Angie just tore me apart. But, as we turned into our road, Angie once again pulled herself together. 'Look, Mill,' she said, furiously drying her face with the back of her hand, 'let's not tell the younger children just yet. We have to tell the older boys, but let's leave it for as long as possible with the little ones, okay? I can't bear for them to know. It won't help them, will it? They'll just be so frightened. We can't tell them. We *can't*.'

I told her yes, and then she took my hand as we pulled up outside our house. 'Look,' she said again, turning to face me, 'if there really is nothing they can do for me – if all they can do is give me chemo to help me live for a little bit longer – then I want to enjoy the time I have left, okay? Carry on as normal, as much as possible, anyway. This cancer might be going to take my life, but it's not going to ruin whatever time I have left, okay?'

We clung together then, before going into the house. I couldn't speak. I thought I'd choke. I couldn't stop sobbing. 'Mill,' Angie said finally, pulling back and looking at me sternly. 'Mill, come on. Pull yourself together, will you? *Please* don't let the children see you looking like this.' She gently wiped the tears off my cheeks with her hands, then looked past me. 'Come on, Mill,' she said. I turned around and looked. And could see that my brothers Barry and Malc were walking down our path, Malc's wife Eileen behind them. And right away I could see we wouldn't have to tell them our devastating news. They could already see by the expressions on our faces.

We got out of the car, and Eileen walked Angie back inside, while Malc and Barry tried to comfort me out on the pavement. I just couldn't seem to get myself together.

'Come on, Ian,' Malc said, as the girls headed into the house. 'I know it's hard, lad, but try to pull yourself together. Don't let the kids see you like this, please. Come on. For *Angie*.'

I looked at my brothers, desperate to do what Malc was asking, but failing. The thought of losing Angie – of her being ripped away from her children so cruelly young – was just so overwhelming, just too much for me to bear. As we walked towards the house, it was like this huge rage building inside me – against an enemy I could do absolutely nothing about.

I couldn't stop myself. And, before either Barry or Malc could stop me, I punched the wall of the house as hard as I could. It didn't make me feel even the tiniest bit better.

*

I was dreading telling the boys. How do you even begin having that sort of conversation – particularly as I was finding it so hard to hold myself together? But Angie wanted it done, I could see that. So, while Malc, Eileen and Barry entertained the younger ones in the living room, we called Reece, Ryan and Damon down into the kitchen. In fact, it all happened in something of a blur after that. Reece came in first, while I was preoccupied trying to hide my bleeding hand from Angie. Before I'd even really composed myself fully, Angie already had her arms around him, telling him. And when the other two came down, clearly confused and upset by what they were seeing, I took them straight out into the garden – to tell them the most devastating news they would ever hear. It was one of the saddest days of my life.

'How long has she got?' Ryan asked me, his eyes pooled with tears. I hadn't seen him cry in such a long time, and it killed me. Damon too. I could see he was incapable of speech, but trying so hard to keep things together.

But it was pointless even to try now, so I gathered them close to me and we cried. And, as we did so, I looked out towards the end of the garden, the garden that was home to the outside members of our extended family. There was Jade's rabbit, Snowdrop, and our two beautiful Harris hawks, Taz and Jess.

Taz was Reece's, Jess was mine – and they had become something of a preoccupation for both of us. Having persuaded Angie of the benefits of Reece's adopting such an outdoorsy hobby, I'd built a big aviary the previous autumn, at the end of the garden, and swiftly caught the same bug myself. The birds needed to fly daily, and we'd go out together to exercise them – tramping over the moors and through the woods near our home, with both of them flying free above our heads. They were wonderful pets; so wild, yet so loyal. They would always come back when we called them.

I could see them now, and hear them calling to us, such a piercing, mournful sound, as if wondering, since we were home, why we hadn't taken them out yet; as if trying to restore a status quo that was no more and could never be returned to. Our lives had changed forever now.

'Oh, Mill,' Angie said to me that night in bed, 'how'd you do that?' She'd seen my scabbed and swollen knuckles, which were hurting really bad now. She took my hand and turned it this way and that, wincing. 'It looks so *painful.*'

'It's nothing,' I said, flexing and unflexing my fingers. 'I just tripped up on the steps earlier when I was out feeding the birds.'

She seemed to accept this and I was glad because I felt terrible for having done it. She needed me right now, and I needed to be strong for her – not saddle her with having to worry about me.

Chapter 9

Ella's party is small – just close family. But, though it goes really well, I know it'll be a bittersweet memory, because every aspect of it is now overlaid by this sense of finality. Will this be the last birthday cake Angie ever bakes for her? The last time she watches her open her birthday presents? The last time she'll get to tell her to make a wish when she blows out her birthday candles, all the while knowing such a horrible truth? Because the truth is that, if Ella was old enough to know what was happening, her one wish would be to have her mummy there to raise her. A wish that's not going to be granted. It must be torture.

I keep thinking back to when Ella opened the parcel containing the little dog, and how the tears were running down Angie's cheeks. But I know I have to stop it. She needs me to be strong. And also capable, if I'm to have any chance of convincing her we'll be okay without her. Which is why I have to concentrate on what she wants to teach me.

I'm learning to do the ironing now, and I'm actually getting good at it. Which is something of a shock as I'm a complete beginner. Angie's always done the ironing, and, because I would never have had a clue where to start, on the rare occasion when Angie wasn't around and I needed a shirt doing, I'd just nip down the road and our Eileen would do it for me. But now I'm getting there. But I have had my moments. I've stuck a pair of Connor's school trousers to the iron, and, worse than that, I've ironed straight over a plastic transfer on one of Jake's T-shirts. Cleaning that off the sole plate took ages. But I'm getting there. I now almost understand the complicated relationship that exists between the dial, the 'shot of steam' button and the creases.

It's no wonder I'm improving, because Angie now makes me iron almost everything. She started off leaving half the ironing pile for me to finish, but now she has me do almost all of it. The art of plaiting hair, however, still eludes me. It's hard plaiting hair. Don't ever let anyone tell you differently. So it's no wonder that I'm having difficulty mastering it. But then, one day, Angie has a brilliant brainwave.

'I tell you what,' she says to me one night when we're sitting in front of the telly. 'I know what we can do. We can practise with my wig.'

It's such a brilliant idea that I'm surprised neither of us has already thought of it. She leaps off the sofa, all pleased with herself, and goes to fetch it from its box in the bedroom. It's been stored there since her hair all grew back again.

'You're not going to put it on, are you?' I ask her, when she bounces back in with it. She also has a brush and comb and a couple of hair bobbles.

'Don't be daft!' she says, laughing. 'Of course not. How would that work? I can't teach you when the thing's on my head, can I? No,' she says, sitting down beside me again. 'Budge up and lift your leg up for me.'

I raise my right leg up a little, not understanding what she's aiming at. And then I realise what her plan is, because she slips the wig snugly over my knee.

'There you are,' she says. 'You're all set.'

'Set for what?' I say, laughing, as I smooth the soft hair down over the leg of my jeans.

'Set to show me if you're getting any better, of course! Because I don't just want you plaiting,' she says. 'I want you *French*-plaiting by the time I've finished with you.'

I shake my head. I don't even know what French-plaiting is. Something to do with frogs' legs? Strings of onions? I just can't picture it. It all gets more complex by the minute.

I suppose there isn't a person alive who, when bad things happen, doesn't think, why me? Hearing the news that Angie's cancer was terminal was one of those times in my life, and, for a while after being told about the secondaries in her lung, I walked round in a fog of such intense anger and distress that it was all I could do to function normally. Why me? I couldn't stop thinking in those terms. Why us? Why all our children – why should *they* be the ones to lose their mother? But, most of all, why her? Why my beautiful Angie? A woman who'd never done a single bad thing in all her life. If there was a God, then how could he do this to her?

I had to be there for Angie and the kids – that went without saying. But for the first couple of days I felt that I wanted to run as far away as possible. That, or just lie down and die myself. I was falling apart, and the tears kept on threatening to spill over. That second day – all of us still shell-shocked – we had Damon over, with Warren and Natalie, and, even though we were talking about something completely unrelated, I found myself overcome with an unstoppable urge to cry.

Not wanting either Angie or Natalie to see me sobbing, I fled the room. Then, conscious of the kids around and not knowing quite where to go, I went outside and climbed into my car. I had no plan on going anywhere – I just needed to try to pull myself together. But after a couple of minutes I was jolted by the vibration of my mobile phone, which was sitting in my lap.

It was my brother, Barry. 'Hey, Ian,' he said. 'I was just calling to see if you're okay.'

I told him I was, but he could obviously tell that I wasn't, from the sound of my broken voice.

'Where are you?' he wanted to know.

I wiped my eyes with my hand. 'Sitting in my car on the drive.'

'Right,' he said. 'I'm coming down to see you right now.'

'No,' I said. 'You can't. I can't have Angie know I've been sitting out here in this state.'

'Then you come straight round here,' he said. 'Fifteen minutes, mind. If you're not here in fifteen minutes, I'll be up there ringing your doorbell, you understand?'

So I went. I drove to Brierley, where they lived, only a mile or so up the road from me. And when I pulled up he and his wife Lynn were already on the doorstep waiting for me. I'd tried to compose myself, but just seeing them both there set me off all over again.

'Why?' I sobbed, holding my arms out in front of them. 'Why my Angie?' I was in such a state by now that I sank to my knees right there in front of them.

They took me inside and did their best to calm me down and console me, though it was obviously hard for them. What do you say to someone in that position? What can you do to make it better?

'I can't believe how much bad luck you've had,' Barry said to me. 'You really were dealt a bad hand, lad.'

To which there seemed nothing to say. I felt so bleak. So helpless. There was nothing I could do to solve this. Nothing anyone could do.

Except be there for us, and I was lucky to have such a supportive family. And after an hour or so of talking, and a couple of mugs of tea, I felt strong enough to go back and face my life again.

'And look, lad,' Barry said as I was leaving, 'we're here for you all. So if you need anything – anything at all – you just ask, okay?'

I said I would. And then even managed a smile, thinking about what my brother had just said to me. Barry's always done well for himself: he's worked hard down the pits for years, and been careful with his money. In fact it's something of a family joke, how careful Barry is with money, and everyone's always pulled his leg about it.

'Okay, Baz,' I said. 'Lend us a thousand quid, then, will you?'

Barry just smiled. 'No, mate, I meant anything. But not money.' Then his expression changed. 'No, even money. Just let me know, mate.'

And it didn't matter that this was one thing money probably couldn't solve, either. It was just the principle. Having a family. That meant the world to me.

But, whatever I would have to come to terms with once Angie had left us, the future was something I had to put out of my mind. It was the here and now that mattered. It was Angie that mattered. We had to make the best of whatever time she had in any way we could.

And chemotherapy, however horrible, could give her some time. I hung onto that. But there would be a cost, and this time it would be a bigger one.

Because Angie was given only radiotherapy after her mastectomy, she didn't lose her hair when she first had breast cancer. But this time it would be different because she was going to have drugs that would not only knock out the cancer cells, but take all her hair off as well.

It broke my heart to know she was going to have to go through that. She'd always had such beautiful hair, and had always taken such good care of it. It started happening right away, too: as soon as she'd finished her second dose of chemo she began noticing that, every time she brushed it, more and more of it would be left in the brush.

'It's finally happening,' she said to me one morning. 'I'm losing it, Mill. I can't be doing with it. Tell you what: let's pop round to our Neil's tonight, and have Diane cut some of it off.'

Neil's Diane was a hairdresser. Had been ever since she left school. She worked in a salon in Barnsley called Lesley Francis. She and Angie were very close, and shared the same sense of humour. And I knew she'd be strong enough to deal with the situation without getting herself in a state about it.

And I was right. We had Reece mind the little ones with his girlfriend Sophie, and when we drove round to Neil and Diane's I could tell Angie already felt better, now she'd made the decision to have some hair off.

While the girls got on with Angie's haircut in the kitchen, Neil and I were in the other room, watching TV. Or, at least, trying to. They were laughing so much that in the end we went to join them to see what was so funny.

We walked in to see Angie, with such a grin on her face, holding a brush that was full of her glossy brown hair. It was heartbreaking to see, but, at the same time, awe-inspiring. Here she was, holding half her hair in her hand, and still managing to keep her sense of humour. 'Look at that,' she said, laughing that big, infectious laugh of hers, 'I'll be bald by the time you take me home, Mill!'

I was awed by my wife that night. And also humbled by her incredible strength and courage. So the next day I decided that, if she was going to have to lose that beautiful hair of hers, then it was my duty to try to make it as painless as possible. She already had a wig: they'd given her one at the hospital. But it was dull and looked synthetic and I knew she hated the thought of wearing it.

She would have just got on with it, though, because that's what she was like, and I also knew that, if I told her what I was up to, she'd just tell me not to be so daft and waste loads of money. So, while she was out visiting her mum, I secretly dug out a photo of her and then took myself off into Barnsley.

I'd done my research on the Internet, so it didn't take too long to find the wig shop. And it looked like just the place. I gave the assistant the photo, which showed Angie's colour and style. 'Have you got one exactly like this?' I asked her. 'It has to be made out of real hair, mind.'

She went away and came back with one that would do the job perfectly – though at a price: it cost £280. But it was just what she needed, and it was worth every penny, just for the look on her face when I brought it home and she opened the box. Her eyes lit up and she gasped. It was as if Christmas had come early. 'Oh, it's beautiful, Mill.' Then she looked concerned. 'But can we afford it? It must have cost you a fortune!'

I shook my head. 'Hundred pounds, that's all.'

Her eyes widened. 'Really?' She picked it up and stroked it. Then her eyes narrowed again. 'Come on, Mill. *Really*?'

It was no good. I couldn't keep it up. Not while I was looking at that expression. So I confessed. 'Oh, Mill,' she said, putting her arms round me and kissing me. 'You really do think a lot of me, don't you?'

It didn't need answering that, not really, but I did anyway. 'Course I do,' I told her. 'And always will.'

Almost all Angie's hair was gone just a few weeks later, but she was ready. She'd had Diane's daughter Jane – also now a hairdresser – cut and style the wig so it looked exactly how she wore her own hair, so that, with her wig on, you'd not have known she was even ill. And the chemo didn't seem to be getting to her either. It was the other way around. Before the chemo she'd also been suffering from something called Horner's syndrome, where one of her eyes had almost closed because of a tumour pressing on a nerve. But that had gone, as well as her breathlessness, and she'd started gaining weight as well. Within a few months, when she had her wig on, you'd never have even known she was terminal. She wasn't tired, didn't seem down – in fact, she was as full of life as ever, running around after the kids as usual, which, given we had so many – not to mention one being a ten-month-old baby – was quite a feat in itself. And there were times when thoughts of the future would seem to disappear into the background. I could go hours sometimes forgetting about the cancer that was killing her. How could someone so full of life be dying?

But it was her humour, most of all, that both humbled and amazed me. Angie was soap mad – always had been, from *Dallas* right up to *Emmerdale* – so there weren't a lot of nights that didn't involve her being glued to one of them. On this night, we were enjoying a chance to watch *Coronation Street*. Connor was upstairs, playing on his beloved Xbox, and Reece had gone out with his mate Benji, up to his farm up the road.

Reece and I had just got back in from flying and feeding the birds. You kept them hungry all day so that they'd come back when you flew them – after the piece of meat you held out for them in your gloved hand. They'd been great pets, but

I'd just made the decision to sell them. Reece was getting older now, more involved with his busy social life, and, with everything else that was happening, I just didn't have the heart or the time to commit to it any more. I needed to focus all my time and attention on Angie and the kids now.

Which meant watching *Coronation Street* with her – though, with the little ones all asleep, I was thinking she maybe had other plans, because she slipped her hand into mine and kept giving me suggestive little smiles.

'Mill,' she said softly, as the adverts came on. 'D'you fancy doing me a little favour?'

I turned to face her and raised my eyebrows at her, equally suggestively.

Angie burst out laughing. '*No*, stupid, not *that* sort of favour! I want you to go and wash my hair for me, while I watch the rest of *Corrie*.'

I blinked at her, confused, not understanding what she was on about. Not, that is, till she suddenly whipped off her wig, and plopped it unceremoniously in my lap.

It sat there, splayed out, like some dead furry animal. Angie roared; she laughed so much she had tears rolling down her cheeks. 'It's all right, this!' she managed to splutter, once she'd regained enough composure. 'You can even wash my hair while I sit and watch TV, and finish off this box of Ferrero Rocher and my cuppa!'

Chemotherapy, however, has a habit of catching up with you, as anyone who's taken it will probably tell you. Though it had seemed for so long that Angie was sailing through her treatment, there came a point when it became obvious she wasn't. I was back from Herbert's one morning, having dropped all the kids off at school, when I came in to hear the sound of her being sick. I rushed up to see her bent over the bathroom sink, vomiting. Retching and retching, she was, trying to hold back her hair. I put my hand on her back and rubbed it till she was done.

'Oh, love,' I said, concerned. 'Are you okay now?'

It was the wrong thing to say. 'Do I *look* okay?' she snapped at me, rising from the sink and turning to round on me. She looked awful. Her skin was grey and clammy, her eyes bloodshot, her cheeks smeared with tears. No, I thought. Of *course* she's not okay. She's dying.

Her shoulders slumped then, as she saw my expression. It wasn't in Angie's nature to snap at anyone. She sighed a heavy sigh and reached for some toilet roll to wipe her face. 'No,' she said. 'No, I'm not. I feel awful.' She sat down on the edge of the bath, the tears rolling down her face. 'I feel terrible. It's the chemo. I know it's doing me good, but I just feel so horrible. So sick and so weak and so *horrible*, Mill.'

'I know, love,' I said. 'But it'll soon be over with now, won't it? How many cycles do you have left now? Two?' I went and sat down beside her, put my arm round her and squeezed her shoulder. 'And when you've finished,' I said, 'you'll feel *so* much better, won't you?'

It was the wrong thing to say again, because her expression was still so angry. 'No, I *won't*, Mill!' she said, her eyes blazing. 'I might not be throwing up, but I certainly won't feel better. Because I won't *be* better, will I? It's not like it's going to cure me, is it? It's just going to slow down me getting *worse*. Just give me a bit more time, Mill. That's all!'

She jerked up then, and reached up to the top of her head, pulled her wig off and threw it angrily at the floor. Then she looked in the mirror, and then looked at my face reflected in it. 'Look at me, Mill!' she shouted at me. '*Look at me!* Look what it's doing to me! I feel awful and I look awful, too! Do you have any idea how I feel when I look at myself in the mirror? *Do* you? I hate it. I hate it. *I hate it!*

I had no idea what to do, so I just gathered her into my arms, and held her there till she stopped crying, and told her that to me she still looked beautiful, that she would *always* look beautiful, and that she was being so brave and so strong that I loved her more than ever. That I loved her, I loved her, I loved her. I just didn't know what else to say.

Later, in the kitchen, when Angie was composed again and able to stomach a cup of tea, I remembered our Terry telling me about his wife Diane's friend, Jean. Like Angie, she'd had breast cancer and had had lung secondaries, too, and he'd been telling me how well she'd been doing since she'd finished her chemo, how she was back out, going down the pub and going on day trips and everything, and how, despite being in her seventies and terminal, she felt so well.

He'd been telling me, I think, to try to reassure *me* about the future, but it occurred to me that maybe she could have a chat with Angie. Perhaps it would perk her up if she could see the light at the end of the tunnel. I was terrified that, if she couldn't see that light, she might just give up.

I called in to see Diane the same afternoon, before I picked the kids up, and she called Jean then and there to fix up for her to pop round the following day.

'Oh, Mill,' Angie said, when I got home and explained about Jean visiting. She shook her head and sighed. 'What are you *like*?'

But I was glad I did, because, when Jean came, she really did look to be doing well, and, listening to them chatting, I could see that Angie was reassured by it, too.

At least I hoped so – she always kept her pain inside so much, did Angie. I just hoped so. I didn't know what else to do for her.

Chapter 10

With the kids back in school now, and Reece gone to work, Angie and I return to hospital to see the oncologist. With Ella's birthday over, we're already into July, and in a couple of weeks the schools will break up for the summer holidays. Our own holiday feels like such a long time ago now, and I try not to think about how quickly the last three months have flown by. There are no more birthdays till my own in October, and then Jade's and Jake's at the end of November. Please God, I think, *please* let Angie be there for the twins' birthday.

It's busy when we arrive at the hospital, and we resign ourselves to a bit of a wait. And, while we do so, Angie gets chatting to the woman sitting next to her. Like Angie, she's a cancer patient, there with her husband, who, when I get chatting to him, turns out to be an ex-miner, like me.

They're an older couple, but her situation's a little like Angie's. The only difference is that her cancer's no longer stable; the disease has once again got the upper hand. 'So they want to give me more chemotherapy,' I hear her telling Angie. 'But I'm not going to. I can't face going through it all again. It just makes me so ill, and at this stage I'd rather have quality of life than quantity.'

Angie's nodding. 'You do wonder if it's worth it,' she agrees. 'Losing all your hair again and feeling sick all the time, and always being so *tired* . . . Maybe it's better to have a bit more quality time, even if overall you get less of it, I suppose.' She seems to think for a second. 'Only the thing is, I've got to think of the children,' she says, sighing. 'I've got a lot of kids and I have to take everything they offer me so I can stay with them as long as possible.'

It's so hard to listen to this, to have to think the unthinkable about what's just around the corner for us. To think about Angie having to go through the slog of chemo again. But, at the same time, the thought of giving up, of giving in, to this wretched, wretched illness . . . And it's an illness that seems to be winning the battle with Angie, too.

I try to keep my fears to myself – try to keep positive about how long she's got – but the truth is that the weight is dropping off Angie now. She won't have it – in fact, she gets cross every time I mention it – but she seems to be fading away in front of me. So much so that, though it's causing such friction between us, I can't help but remark on it – and often do.

So when we go in, and the oncologist says he's pleased with her scan, I'm really shocked. And, when he adds that she seems to be stable at the moment, I refuse to believe it. Yes, it's what I want to hear, but it's so at odds with what I'm seeing that I can't just sit there and say nothing, particularly when he starts telling her that he'll see her again in three months. Three *months*?

'But she's clearly *not* stable,' I point out. 'Look at her! Why can't you look at the scans *and* the patient? She's lost so much weight. Everyone can see that.'

The oncologist turns to Angie. 'Do you think that's so?' he asks her.

I can sense the tension in the air and catch Angie's look. It's a look that's telling me I shouldn't have raised my voice. 'Yes,' she agrees calmly. 'I have lost a bit. But I think it's because I've stopped eating so much junk food. I feel fine in myself.'

I can't argue with both of them, and I don't want to upset Angie, especially because, deep down, I know why she's saying this: it's because, despite what I heard her say to the woman in the waiting room, she's actually not keen on putting herself through more chemo. And who am I to insist? It's her life.

I'm also sure – even though I dare not bring it up now – that she knows just how ill she is but is trying to keep it from us all, so she doesn't cause us even more distress.

I feel despair snapping at my heels as we walk back to the car. She's dying before my eyes and I feel powerless to stop it – surely there's *something* that can be done?

It wasn't just Angie's hair that was to fall victim to her disease. More brutally, her teeth were at risk too. Because the cancer was also in her bones now, in the November of 2008 it was decided that she was eligible to be entered into a clinical trial of a new drug that targeted bone cancer, called Zometa. The only snag, the surgeon explained when we went for an appointment to assess things, was that if she had any teeth that were loose – and it seemed she did have one – then the only way they could give her the drug would be if she had all of them removed first. The alternative was stark: yes, it might give her more time, but she'd spend it with agonising toothache.

Angie was devastated. Losing her hair was one thing, but the prospect of losing her teeth was quite another, and the idea of it really upset her. 'Oh, God, Mill,' she said, late that night, as it had begun to sink in. 'I'm going to look a right state, aren't I? No teeth. No hair. It's like this cancer's just taking me away a bit at a time, isn't it?' But, for once, there was no accompanying smile. She wasn't making light of it. As soon as she said it, she burst into tears.

I pulled her close and tried to console her, told her how much I wished we could change places. Tried to point out that losing her teeth might be horrible to have to go through, but, if it kept her with us for a bit longer, then, to me, it would be worth it. 'And besides,' I tried to joke, 'your new teeth will be perfect. You'll have a Hollywood smile – people pay thousands for one of them.'

But though she dried her eyes and nodded, and would make the best of it when it came to it, I knew we were both crying inside.

She did get a stay of execution, though. It was decided to postpone the trial till they were clearer about the potential benefits, but, as we waited, I kept coming back to the same distressing fact: that the drugs that would cause her so much trauma and pain weren't even going to save her life. Surely there must be something out there that might?

By this time we'd heard about the patient liaison officers (PALS) at the hospital. We'd gone to see them because at our latest appointment, which was with a doctor in the chest clinic, Angie's scans showed that one of her lung tumours had shrunk down really small and he asked us if we'd considered having it taken out.

What he'd said made no sense to us at all. We'd already been told there was no point in Angie having her lung tumour removed – was this doctor telling us something different? There was so much complicated science in all this and we were both beginning to get so confused. Did he know something the oncologist didn't?

PALS are there to support patients and their families while they are undergoing treatment, and offer general advice about any matters relating to the medical process, as well as being able to act as a patient's voice: they can make a note of questions the patient wants to ask their doctors, and go into consultations with them. In this way they can both ask the questions patients might forget if they got emotional or flustered and help explain the answers afterwards.

It was an emotional meeting, as we'd just had the news about the tumour, and I'd got my hopes up again that perhaps something could be done for Angie, and having it brought home to me again that there was nothing that could be done that would actually stop her dying – tumour or no tumour – was another real body blow. But the officer who spoke to us, Lynne Handley, was kind and really helpful.

We explained the situation, and about Angie's cancer being terminal, and, as we did so, I could feel myself getting really upset. 'How will I cope?' I asked her tearfully. 'How will I manage without her? How on earth will I be able to raise all our kids on my own? I'm a man! I don't have a clue. We've been together since we were only kids ourselves!'

I could tell Lynne didn't know what to say to this outburst. But she didn't need to speak, because Angie did. 'You mean you won't have anyone to do the washing-up for you,' she said quietly. She took my hand and squeezed it reassuringly. 'So you might have to get a dishwasher, Mill, that's all.' She smiled at me. 'Or maybe some rubber gloves?'

Which made me feel silly, but also a lot better. And having someone like Lynne to talk to was really comforting as well, as she said she'd be happy to go through Angie's medical notes with me, which made me feel we had someone to support us.

So it was to Lynne that I first went when, a few weeks after our first meeting, I had something that potentially might save Angie. It was an article about the American actor Patrick Swayze that I'd found on the Internet. He had undergone a treatment in Stanford University, in the USA – something called 'cyber knife' radiotherapy. It was an experimental treatment in which radiation was delivered with pinpoint precision, without damaging the surrounding tissue. The only problem, with this not being available in Britain, was how to find the £35,000 or so needed to get it for Angie.

'Take my money,' my mum said. 'I've got fifty thousand

pounds just sitting there in the bank, Ian. Take it all and save Angie's life.'

It was such an amazing gesture and I could never thank Mum enough for it. Or the rest of my family, as it turned out, since the money – which was compensation for the coal dust that took my dad's life far too early – was cash that my mother had always refused to spend. It was our inheritance, she'd always told us, so she would never spend a penny of it. Yet here she was now, along with all my siblings, wanting to give it to me, to get Angie well.

But our hopes were dashed anyway. It would be wasted on such a treatment. Though Lynne listened to me patiently while I showed her all my cuttings and explained the treatment, she held out little hope that it would help. And, once we went in for Angie's consultation, the oncologist confirmed it. 'It would make no difference,' she explained patiently. 'This is a treatment that's been used on lung-cancer patients, which isn't what Angie's got. She has breast cancer that's now spread to the lung, which is different.'

I was devastated. And very distressed. So Lynne asked the oncologist to explain why that made it different. 'Because if it were lung cancer,' she explained, 'and the whole lung was removed, there would be a good chance that the cancer would have gone with it. But this is cancer that has already spread around Angie's body. And is also already in her bones.'

By now I was sobbing freely. I couldn't stop myself. I'd allowed myself to hope again, and now that hope had been taken away from me. It didn't matter how much money Mum had. It wouldn't work.

'Mill,' Angie was whispering to me, stroking my hand. 'You have to accept that there's nothing anyone can do now.'

Something snapped in me then, and I shrugged off her hand. 'I will never accept that!' I shouted. 'I will never give up, *never*!'

The room fell silent. And it was only then that I realised how upset everybody was as a result of my shouting. Lynne was speaking to me now. 'Ian,' she said. 'Why don't you both come down to my office for ten minutes? Take time to compose yourself. I can't have you going home like this.'

I could see Angie was really upset as well, and also keen to do that, so I nodded and followed them out of the doctor's office. Once again, it was I who had to pull myself together, I thought wretchedly, while Angie conducted herself so bravely. I felt terrible.

But I was soon going to feel even more terrible. I stopped in the cloakrooms to splash some water on my face, saying I'd be there in a moment or two, but when I got down to the PALS office, Angie immediately leapt up, saying she needed to go and get herself a drink.

'I'll get it for you,' I said, keen to try to make amends for what had happened.

'No, Mill,' she said. 'I'll get it. I need the walk.'

As soon as she'd gone, Lynne sat me down, then sat opposite. 'Ian, I'm so sorry the outcome of the meeting isn't what you'd hoped for,' she said gently. She then paused. 'But, Ian, there's something else I need to say to you. Angie's tired. And she's worried that she hasn't got loads of time left. And what time she *has* got she wants to share with you and the children.'

I felt the tears prickling at my eyes again. 'Lynne, are you asking me to give up on Angie?'

'I would never ask that of you, Ian,' she said. 'I'm asking you to give her what she most needs at this time.' She paused. 'Which is her loving husband's *time* back.'

There was nothing I could say to that. It hit me like a punch in my chest. They had obviously spoken, and Angie had obviously asked Lynne to make that point to me. 'I'll try,' I said dejectedly. 'I promise. I will really try.'

But it was so hard. Every fibre of my being railed against it. If there was anything I could do to save her, then I'd do it. And, despite the promise I'd just made to Lynne Handley, I told Angie exactly that as we got into the car: that I refused to just accept she was going to die.

She rounded on me immediately. 'Mill, you *have* to!' she fumed at me. 'Because that's what's going to happen!' I couldn't remember the last time I'd seen her so angry with me.

But I was equally angry with her. 'Why would I do that? And why are you so cross?' I shouted, feeling furious as well now. 'How can you just sit there accepting you're going to die? What about us? What about me and the kids? At least I'm *trying*! At least I'm doing something instead of nothing!'

'But I *am* thinking of you and the kids, Mill! And me as well! I have so little time left to be with you all – are you going to waste all of it running around looking for cures when there isn't one? Is that how you want to spend what time we have left? Because I don't! D'you understand? *I don't!*

We drove home in silence. Well, virtual silence. I was so angry that I shouted at every junction at every car that got in my way. And every time I raised my voice I could feel Angie's eyes burning into me. Then she'd silently shake her head and look away.

When we got home I slammed the car door as hard as I could and stormed into the house, still fuming.

My brother Glenn was there, with Ella, and must have been mortified to find himself in the middle of it all.

And he was definitely in the middle of it all at that moment. 'Do you want a cuppa while I'm making one, or what?' I snapped at Angie.

Glenn looked at me. 'What's up, Ian?' he said mildly. 'They haven't given you more bad news at the hospital, have they?'

'No,' I said. 'It's *her*. She just seems to've thrown the towel in.'

Angie looked at me, and her voice was as calm as mine was heated. 'No, I haven't, Mill. I just don't want you spending hours and hours on that computer looking for cures when there isn't one. You keep building your hopes up for nothing and you're going to make yourself ill too.'

'How do you know?' I rounded on her. 'How do you know there isn't a cure out there somewhere? There's all sorts of clinical trials out there – and even the scientists don't know if one of them might cure cancer. That's why they have them! And, even if it doesn't cure it, it'll at least give me some hope when there isn't any! What if it was me? If it was me with cancer would *you* just sit back and accept it?'

Angie didn't speak. She just looked at me. And I could see Glenn was looking at me, too. I'd said my piece but what could they say in response to it? Clearly nothing. So I stomped off into the kitchen to make the tea.

It was while I was in there, pouring it out, feeling really guilty now for having shouted, that Angie came up behind me, put her arms around my waist and pressed her face against my back. 'No, Mill,' she whispered. 'You're right. If I were you, I wouldn't be able to accept it either. I know I couldn't.'

Chapter 11

My mum died on 13 September 2009. She was eighty-seven, so she'd had a long life, and, mostly, I think, a happy one. Not that it wasn't hard (she brought eight kids up without microwaves or washing machines, and did it well), but, though she'd lost my dad almost twenty years earlier, she'd never lost her energy. With us all being so close, we'd most of us stop by every day, and you'd never find her sitting doing nothing. She used to have my niece Jane – Karen's daughter – round to do her hair for her every month, and was always up for it when Terry or I suggested a day trip out shopping.

Though you always have it in your mind that your parents aren't going to live forever, it was no less of a shock when Glenn came banging on our front door at one that morning, and shouting through the letterbox to come quick because they thought she'd had a stroke.

Mum lived at the bottom of our street – she and Dad had moved in when the houses were first built – but I knew the chances were that she'd be straight off to hospital. So, once I'd thrown some clothes on, I drove back down with Glenn to wait for the ambulance – and, as it was just leaving by then, with both her and my brother Les in it, I joined a convoy of all my other brothers following behind.

We met my sister Karen and her husband at the hospital – my poor sister was sobbing her heart out – and it didn't take long for the doctors to assess the situation. Mum had definitely had a stroke, they said, and it had also been a big one. She wouldn't regain consciousness, and we should all prepare for the worst.

And the worst happened only half a day later. Mum was taken up to the cancer ward, the same one Angie used to go to for her chemo – Ward 24. Mum died there at eleven the following morning. We were all with her, taking it in turns to hold her hand and stroke her hair, hair that was soft and shoulder-length, and still grey – it hadn't even gone fully white. And they gave her the best care imaginable. Even though she'd never know anything about it, she died with such dignity, and I could never thank the nurses on that ward enough. Even though she was unconscious, and not in pain, they still looked after her so lovingly, wiping her face, plumping her pillows, smoothing her hair.

It was devastating to lose her so suddenly, and not having the chance to say goodbye, but, if such things are possible, Mum's was a good death, one that was surrounded by people who loved her and cared for her – a fitting reflection of all the love and care she'd always given us.

Mum's on my mind today, for some reason. It's been over a year since she passed away now and the time's gone so quickly, and thinking that leads me straightaway to thinking about time generally. How much does Angie have of it? Will it go that fast too?

We're off to the dental hospital in Sheffield this morning, Angie and I, while Glenn stays at ours to look after the children. In the end it was decided that Angie could enter the trial for Zometa, so, finally – a whole year after the wheels were put in motion to make it happen (not to mention several reminders from her doctor) – Angie's appointment to have her teeth out has come through.

It's a drive of around fifteen miles and a journey neither of us has been looking forward to. And Angie's very quiet, not at all her usual talkative self. Finally, she sighs. 'I'm dreading this, Mill,' she tells me. 'I just want it done. I wish it was *already* done. I'm really dreading it.'

I feel so sad for her. She's already been through so much, and now this. And though I know being on Zometa might give her a little more time with us, having all her teeth out will be so traumatic. I find myself beginning to understand Angie's ambivalence about enduring further treatment. Who would want to be put through such a grisly thing?

But, as if that weren't bad enough, we get to the hospital only to be told that they can't provide her with any dentures. She will have to go to our own dentist and get some made up – a process that could take several weeks. I am appalled and Angie, always so strong, is close to tears.

'What, you mean . . . ?' she gasps, as what the dental surgeon says begins to sink in. 'You're going to take all my teeth out, and leave me with *nothing*?' she splutters, and I hear the exasperation in her voice. 'You mean I just have to walk out of here without a tooth in my head?' She spreads her palms in astonishment, tears glinting in her eyes. 'But how am I supposed to even eat?'

The dentist is apologetic, and says we should have been told about having to get some dentures made up ready, but I feel frustrated. Nobody *did* say, so how were we supposed to know? He suggests we go away and do that and then they can make us a new appointment, but I tell him we won't bother – we've already waited a year for this one, after all, and if our own dentist is going to make up the dentures, we might as well have him pull Angie's teeth as well.

And that's it. All that stress Angie's had to go through for nothing. And is now going to have to go through all over again. We stop off at our own dentist on the way home.

The business of Angie's teeth is really getting to both of us. Though it's clearly necessary, it feels so brutal – almost like an act of violence – and, now she finally has some dentures being prepared for her, I know it's really playing on her mind.

Mindful of how hard it must be for her to remain so strong for the children, I make a real effort to keep the mood light. I know I must do things the way *she* wants them done: to try to live our lives without reference to the cancer that dominates them, but instead as if everything were fine. Because that's what she *does* want – to make every day a special one. Not one in which we stand at odds, with me manning the battlements, grim-faced and desperate and driven, but one that will instead add to the stock of happy memories the children have, to sustain them when she's no longer here.

The following Sunday – and conscious that she's due to have her teeth out, and that eating might soon become a misery, even if only for a time – I decide to cook a roast chicken dinner with all the trimmings.

I have the kitchen to myself on Sunday mornings most weeks these days, in any case, as it's the time when Angie tends to take the younger ones to visit her mum and dad.

Angie's parents are getting elderly now – Herbert's ninety-one and Winnie's eighty-seven. Herbert's incredible for his age, though – fit as a flea. He's very active, and always busy in his garden, either tending to the mass of flowers he grows from seed, or in his greenhouse, looking after his beloved tomatoes.

Winnie's not so good, however. She's becoming frail and keeps having falls. And, as she's weak now, Herbert often phones me (we live only half a dozen houses away from them) so I can give him a hand with putting her to bed.

I'd do anything for Herbert and Winnie. They're like a second mum and dad to me. I can remember back to when Angie and I were courting and how much they accepted me and loved me. I'd go round after a day shift down the pit – I'd always want to go and see Angie before I even went home – and Winnie would always plonk this huge roast dinner in my lap; the biggest roast dinner you ever saw.

With the house quiet for the first time in what seems like days, I get cracking with making mine. Get the chicken in, do all the veg, make all the trimmings. I do it all: roast potatoes, stuffing, three veg, pigs in blankets, Yorkshire puddings – the whole works.

'Who says men can't cook?' I ask Pebbles, who's waiting patiently on the floor beside me, hoping for scraps. I feel ridiculously proud of my efforts. I can't smell it myself, of course – more's the pity – but I love the thought that *they* will, once they all come running back in for their dinner.

And they're starving – they always are – and they can't wait to taste it.

'Wow, Dad, that smells nice!' says Connor, sniffing the air appreciatively.

'Aw, Mill,' adds Angie, popping her head round the dining room door. 'You've laid the table so nicely, too.'

And even little Corey joins in, rubbing his belly and going, 'Yummy yummy in my tummy!' as he always does.

But, when I get everyone seated and everyone begins digging in, Connor immediately pulls a face. 'Dad,' he says, screwing his face up. 'This is *horrid*!'

I look around the table to see other similarly perplexed faces, and as Angie begins hers, one of disgust. Amused disgust, yes, but still disgust.

'Oh, love,' she says, putting her cutlery down. 'This is *curry*. You've made curry sauce instead of gravy.'

We troop back to the kitchen, and she immediately sees the reason for my mistake. There are two canisters in the cupboard – one of Bisto Chicken Gravy, and one of Bisto Chip Shop Curry Sauce. Both canisters are orange, and I have used the wrong one. And, because I have no sense of smell, I've failed to notice my mistake – a mistake that has ruined our perfect Sunday dinner.

It's a costly as well as a dispiriting mistake, too. No one wants to eat it now – even if we *do* scrape all the sauce off, everyone's food is already getting cold. The entire meal ends up in the composting caddy. It fills it to the very brim. It's heartbreaking.

I'm so furious with myself. It's been such a massive waste of effort, and, to cap it all, the children – who are obviously hungry – start squabbling. But, as ever, it's Angie who lightens the situation. She just can't stop giggling about it. Every time she catches my eye she bursts out laughing, so that, by the time I get my car keys and head out to buy more food to cook, even I'm seeing the funny side. God, though, I think as I head off down the road, how the hell am I going to get by without her?

July sees our silver wedding anniversary approaching, and for once I try to forget about my desperate quest for cures, and concentrate on making it special for Angie. It might, after all, be the last wedding anniversary we share.

Having arranged that Ryan and Damon will move back in to help Reece look after the little ones for the weekend, I secretly book us a couple of days in Llandudno, in North Wales. It's a favourite place of ours, and just a few miles down the coast from Rhyl, scene of so many magical holidays in our youth.

We loved going to Rhyl. And so did Angie's parents. They would take their two-week summer holiday there every single year, always booking the same flat, in Edward Henry Street, as well. And, once I met Angie and became part of the family, I would go too. They'd have to book a minibus because there'd be so many of us: Angie's brother Neil, and Diane, her brother Des and his wife, Lynne, her divorced older sister Diane (who'd go on to marry my brother Terry) and her little lad Jonathan – and, of course, us.

And we'd get into a routine, too – Angie's dad would spend the whole day laid out on a towel, sunbathing, by the kids' boating pool, and every lunchtime, after doing the market, Winnie would come and join him, bringing a huge picnic and the biggest flask of coffee I'd ever seen. The rest of us would come and go – Angie and I would mostly be around and about with Neil and Diane – and then at 6 p.m. sharp we'd be back for dinner.

Then it was out for the evening, usually to the Victory Club. It was in the Victory Club that I was first introduced to bingo. And I had some beginner's luck, too – or so I thought – as, in the packed club, I had a full house right away. Except I didn't. I'd misheard and marked off the wrong number. I don't think I'll *ever* forget the embarrassment of hearing the man shout, 'False call!' I was eighteen and just about as red as humanly possible, feeling a right lemon and looking for a mousehole to crawl into. And all the while Angie laughed her head off.

I've never played bingo again.

I don't tell Angie about the anniversary trip till the day before we're going, and she's ecstatic.

'Aw, Mill,' she goes, '*Wow*. And I don't even mind getting lost in Manchester. In fact, it won't be the same if we *don't* get lost in Manchester, will it? Won't be the same if we don't get to see Cheadle!'

You'd think we had a second home in Cheadle, we've been there that many times. We don't seem to be able to go anywhere near Manchester *without* ending up there. It's always been the same, to the great amusement of Angie's dad – right from when I passed my driving test and Angie and I would drive ourselves. We'd go round roundabout after roundabout, but, no matter how good Angie's map reading, I always seemed to be in the wrong lane at the wrong moment, and off we'd head in entirely the wrong direction. And always the *same* wrong direction – as if we had shares in the place.

'Where ya been, lad?' Herbert would chuckle, when we finally arrived, an hour after everyone else had. 'Tha been off visiting Cheadle again?'

Though we can't really afford it, I've decided to go upmarket for our break, and have booked us into the swankiest four-star establishment I could find: the St George's Hotel. And on this occasion, with so little time, I want us to make North Wales without a detour. Amusing though it might have been to revisit Cheadle, I want everything to go smoothly, because this is going to be a special time for us. So I have Angie call her Neil to see if we can borrow his satnav.

'You know what, Mill?' Angie says, when Neil brings it round. 'This is just what you need to get. Just think of all the money we'd have saved in petrol all those years if we'd had one of these. Doesn't bear thinking about, does it?'

I try not to think about not having Angie beside me, navigating (even if we *did* always get lost in Manchester), and, by the time we finally reach North Wales, I manage it. Instead, I'm concentrating on giving Angie the best weekend imaginable, living in the moment, looking forward to really treating her like the princess she is.

And it will be a treat, because I've already been on and booked one. When I made the reservation, they had an offer on: something they called their Summer Sizzler. It's a three-course meal for two, and even includes a pair of cocktails, all for the price of twenty quid. Which seemed a bargain when I ordered it and now seems an even bigger one, given how grand the hotel looks when we pull up. Right on the seafront, it has breathtaking views of the whole bay, and, as we arrive, the sea is sparkling invitingly. The whole place looks so pretty – just like a postcard. 'Oh, Mill,' Angie cries as we walk up the steps of the grand entrance. 'I feel like royalty!'

It's a lovely day, so we stroll to the shops hand in hand. Angie wants to take a look around and buy the kids some presents. And, after a languid stroll back, we're both feeling completely relaxed, and it being our anniversary and everything – and, even more to the point, we're alone for once – we end up in bed.

Not long after, my mobile rings, and I wonder if it's Ryan or Damon – some problem or other with one of the kids. But it's our Terry. 'Ay up, Ian,' he says. 'How's it going down there? Have you had your Summer Sizzler yet?'

I look at Angie beside me. 'Yep,' I tell him, grinning. 'Yep, we've definitely had our Summer Sizzler. And it were bloody great, nip!'

It takes Angie a moment to cotton on. 'Mill!' she says, horrified. 'You're crackers, you! I feel really, *really* embarrassed now! Honestly!' She hauls the blanket over her head, but I can tell she's really laughing.

The smile stays on my face right through dinner.

But it's a happy mood that doesn't last the night. How can it? After our meal, seeing that it's so warm, we decide to take a walk along the prom and, once we've found a bench we like, we sit down to watch the sunset.

And we're not alone. It seems everywhere I look there are other couples strolling. And my eyes can't help but be drawn to all the elderly men and women sitting down on nearby benches, just as we are, or ambling hand in hand along the seafront. And, while I sit, with Angie's head nestled between my arm and my shoulder, I remember all the things we used to say to each other when we were teenagers. How when we were old, and had had our kids and they'd all flown the nest, we'd buy a caravan at Thornwick and go there all the time. How Angie would always giggle, whenever we'd see a little old couple shuffling along arm in arm, and say, 'Can you imagine when we're like that, Mill?'

And it's all gone. It's not for us now. And I feel this terrible ache inside. The pain of knowing that it's never going to happen.

*

The next day, we visit Rhyl, and it seems only to underline the already melancholy tone. The exuberant place we remember with such affection from the seventies – the kaleidoscope of lights from the arcades, the smell of hot dogs and fried onions and the sound of girls screaming coming from the fairground – has become a sad and empty shadow of its former self. The amusement arcades are boarded up, most of the hotels are derelict, and the fairground we couldn't wait to visit – and had such fun in – is now just an overgrown expanse of grass, half hidden behind rusty corrugated sheets.

It sends a chill through both of us, this ghost town, and we decide not to linger. 'This is heartbreaking, isn't it?' Angie says. And I agree with her. I wanted to bring her here so we could rekindle the million happy memories we made. But it hasn't worked. It's just depressing to see the state the place is in. She squeezes my arm. 'Let's go home, shall we, Mill? Let's not hang around here. Ella and Corey'll be wondering what's happened to us by now, won't they? I'd much rather get home and give them their presents.'

And I would too. I no more want to be reminded of the past now than the future. Just want more of the now. We hurry home. To where there's life.

Chapter 12

How much do photos matter in the big scheme of things? Not a lot. Not to most sane people, anyway. A picture might paint a thousand words, and a snap capture a moment, but is looking back at photographs of the past – practising nostalgia – generally helpful? Generally not. Better to try to live life in the present.

But, when someone you love is dying, all that goes out of the window. When you know time's short, and that person won't be around for that much longer, knowing you'll have pictures to look at is a comfort. So, when we arrived in Llandudno and realised we'd forgotten to take the camera, we rushed straight out and bought a couple of disposables instead, so that we could take lots of photos of our anniversary trip.

And Angie's been on at me about picking them up from the photo shop since I dropped them off. So a few days later, after looking in on Herbert, I pop into the shop to collect them. But there's a problem. The girl seems to spend ages trying to find them and, when she comes back to me, she's the bearer of bad news.

'I'm really sorry,' she says. 'But there are no pictures. The films were damaged.'

'Damaged?' I say. 'How? The cameras were fine when we brought them in here.'

She shakes her head. 'No, it was in here that they were damaged. One of our machines was faulty and it ruined both the films. I'm so sorry,' she says again.

My heart sinks. I know Angie will be devastated. I know why, too. The same reason she was so keen to get disposables. So I'd have some pictures to remind me of our twenty-fifth anniversary, when the time comes that she'll no longer be here.

'Were none salvageable?' I ask the girl. 'Was every single one ruined?' And, when she tells me this is the case, I explain that it was our silver wedding, and that Angie's cancer is terminal. Nothing can be done about it, obviously, but, by the time I've finished telling her, she's looking even more upset about it than I am.

'I tell you what we can do,' she says. 'Have you got a special photo you'd like us to blow up for you, maybe? We could do that and put it on canvas for you. Would that help?'

I thank her, but I drive home dreading telling Angie, and when I do so she's every bit as devastated as I expected her to be. The shop's gesture was a nice one, and I'm grateful, and Angie chooses a photo for them to enlarge for us, but, with everything else, couldn't she be allowed that one break? It feels like such a kick in the teeth.

*

I'm braced for more bad news, too, when the beginning of September comes around and Angie's due for her next appointment with her consultant. Every time we visit the hospital now, it feels (to me, at least) as if we're walking into the jaws of a nightmare, expecting the worst, but with every other option now closed to us. When we get there, however, and Angie's been weighed and examined, the doctor surprises me by telling us that there doesn't seem to be much progression.

I try to take this in – square what we're being told with what I'm seeing day to day – but, much as I want to believe it, it makes no sense to me. I've been trying to avoid thinking about it, because it's too upsetting to see it happening, but there's no getting away from the truth any more: my wife is still shrinking before my eyes. Angie's clothes are hanging off her now. She's gone from a size ten to a size six, and she's getting weaker as a result of it. She struggles to pick the little ones up now – especially Corey. And it's obvious why: it's because she hardly eats. I keep bringing it up, telling her that Corey eats more than she does, that all she ever does is nibble; but if I go on too much she just gets annoyed with me. 'Stop going on about it, Mill,' she says. 'I feel fine. Stop all your wittering.' But she's not fine. Anyone can see that. And she *still* has that cough.

But I feel at odds with both Angie and her consultant. Both seem determined to gloss over it – Angie particularly. She keeps playing down her weight loss as if it were perfectly normal, saying she's just stopped eating rubbish, that's all. But I don't buy it – you'd never make this much difference by

IAN MILLTHORPE

leaving out a few bags of crisps here and there. She's *not* eating. And she's not eating because the cancer is eating *her*.

Having the pair of them gang up on me, almost, and her keep trying to explain away her weight loss makes my irritation turn to anger and my anger spill over into fury. 'Can't you see my wife is dying?' I shout at the startled consultant. '*Can't* you? There's got to be *something* you can do!'

I know I've lost it, but their faces tell me I've *really* lost it. Both Angie and the consultant have tears in their eyes now, and there's something else in Angie's – a look of real disgust at my behaviour. I'm mortified now, but I just can't seem to stop myself from railing at them. 'Something's going on,' I persist. 'You need to scan her! Not just sit there and tell me nothing's changed! You need to scan her and find out what's going on!'

The doctor, probably as a result of my raising my voice so much, nods. 'Okay, Mr Millthorpe,' she says finally. 'I will book Angie in for another CT scan in the next few weeks, and will arrange to see her to review it at the beginning of November. But you need to understand that, even if we *do* find there's progression, there's still nothing we can actually do now.' She turns to Angie. 'All we can do is give you drugs to help with any pain. There's no point in considering further chemo at this stage, and even if we did it would only be palliative.'

Angie nods at this. I can see that her head's gone down, that she's just accepting this. And it makes me want to burst into tears myself. Why are they just going to let it keep growing?

But her head hasn't gone down that much, not with me,

126

anyway. She rounds on me as soon as we leave the consultant's office. She is furious.

'How could you do that?' she rails at me as we walk back down the hospital corridor. 'How could you shout at my doctor like that, Mill? How *could* you?' She turns to face me. 'Did you see what you did in there, Mill? *Did* you? She was almost in *tears!*'

I have that by now familiar feeling of remorse. Angie is very close to her oncologist and my behaviour towards her has obviously really upset her. I try to apologise, because the last thing I want is to see Angie crying. But at the same time, even though I'm consumed with guilt for losing my temper in such a way, I still can't accept this is all they can do for her. I just *can't.* I just feel compelled to make them see what I'm seeing – to try *anything*. How can I make myself act any differently? How can anyone let someone they love go without a fight?

I try again in the car on the way home – try to get her to understand why I was out of order. 'Look,' I say. 'I know I did wrong, but it's because I feel I have to. If you didn't keep playing down your symptoms all the time, and told them the *truth* about your weight loss, then I wouldn't end up raising my voice with her, would I? It's only because of that – because I want them to *do* something. How the hell do you expect them to treat you if you keep telling them you're fine when you're not?'

It's a full half a minute before Angie answers.

'I feel *fine*, Mill,' she says quietly, but firmly. 'And they're going to scan me now, anyway. So we'll see, won't we?'

We both lapse into silence. She looks so ill now. So wasted.

And her telling me she feels fine again makes me feel worse. She doesn't *want* anyone to do anything, and that's the end of it as far as she's concerned. And she's still angry with me, I know, as I know she's every right to be, so it's a tense and uncomfortable journey home.

When we get out of the car I try to reach her again. 'Hey, Angie,' I say, smiling. 'You may be only small, but you've certainly got a bloody temper on you, lass.'

She looks at me across the car roof, and smiles her big smile. I know she doesn't want to keep this up any more than I do. She shuts the car door. 'I know you're only thinking about me, Mill, so I'll let you off.' The smile widens. 'After you've made me a cuppa, anyway.'

Once we're indoors, and the tea's made, I telephone Lynne at PALS. She has been so patient and so kind, and such an amazing support to Angie, and, when I explain how upset I am that they seem to have just given up now, she promises she'll look into everything for me, and see if there's any way she can get the scan and the next appointment brought forward.

In the meantime, there's another grim ordeal lined up for Angie, as her dentures are ready and she can now have all her teeth removed. A few days later, the kids at school, I can only look on helplessly as my poor wife has all her teeth extracted. And it's as grim as we'd both feared – and yet another bar to her eating, because every time she tries to she's in agony.

'Christ, Mill,' she says. 'It's like chewing on glass.'

And there's nothing I can do to make it better.

*

True to her word, Lynne manages to get Angie's scan made a priority, and, once it's done, she calls with further good news. The oncologist has agreed to move Angie's appointment forward to 30 September, both to review the result and to answer my questions about further treatment, and explain her reasoning in not giving further chemo.

But fate has another cruel surprise for us before that happens, because on 25 September Angie's mum is taken into hospital, seriously ill, and I feel the cold dread of knowing we're going to lose her.

To lose her lovely mum would be *all* Angie needs at such a terrible time, and I pray so hard that Winnie will pull through. But the signs aren't good, and on the 28th our worst fears are confirmed: we get a call saying that she's taken a turn for the worse, and that it would be best if we all went to the hospital.

As with my own mum, it's quick. Winnie passes away that evening, with the whole family around her bedside, including Herbert, her beloved husband of fifty-seven years and who I worry will now be a broken man.

'Please God,' I hear him whisper as he clutches her lifeless hand. 'Please God. Please just take me too.'

Typically, Angie, though so distraught, is more concerned about her dad. It's one in the morning by the time we get home from the hospital, and everyone is shattered, specially Angie herself. I know the last couple of days have really taken it out of her – physically as well as emotionally. Herbert's gone home now, and, though her brother Desmond went home with him, Angie's still worried about him and wants me to go round and check he's okay. She tells me she just can't bear to think of him going back into their home knowing Winnie's never coming back.

'Can you go and see him, Mill?' she asks me. 'Just to make sure he's okay? I won't get a wink of sleep otherwise, and I know he'll feel so much better for seeing you.'

So I go round, to find Herbert sitting in the living room, in his usual armchair, still and silent, the grief etched so clearly on his face. But he's okay, he reassures me. And I trust that he is. He's a strong man, is Herbert, and I feel better for seeing him too.

Des has already made him a cuppa so he doesn't need anything from me. Except for one thing, and I'm so touched that he should ask it. 'Will you arrange the funeral for me, lad?' he asks. 'I know I can trust you to take care of things. The very best, mind. No matter what the cost is. The very best, lad. Can you do that for me?'

I tell him I'll be honoured to.

As I go to leave I ask him one more time if he's sure he's okay. 'I'm fine, Mill,' he tells me. 'Life has to go on, lad. Go on, go home. Get back to our Angie and the kids.'

As I suspected, Angie's still waiting up for me when I cross the street. 'How's he doing?' she asks as soon as I'm inside. I tell her about arranging the funeral and about what Herbert said to me. And she just smiles, and takes my hand in hers. 'He's right, Mill,' she tells me. 'Life *does* go on.'

And I know it's me she's talking to, as well.

*

Once I've dropped the kids at school and Corey at nursery the next morning, I leave Angie and Ella and go straight to the funeral directors over in Shafton. And I do everything just the way Herbert's told me to – I get the best. I order her the same Last Supper coffin that my own mum was buried in (it's solid oak and it really shines – almost like a mirror) as well as ordering a four-foot cross to sit on top of it, made of white flowers and red roses, and three limousines for the close family to travel in.

And, while I'm there, thoughts of death and dying clamour in my head, obviously. But, though I want to push them away – push back the moment when I have to do this for my Angie – I do have a sudden moment of clarity. Angie's always wanted to be cremated, same as all her siblings, but, like Winnie, I want to be buried. However, there being so many of us in our family, we can't all be buried in the plots by our mum and dad. So we've always agreed that it should be Les and Glenn who have those ones, those two being the ones who have never married.

And now it hits me: I should see if I can buy a plot close to Winnie, so when my time comes I can lie close to her instead. After all, she's been like a second mum to me since I was fourteen years old, and especially since my own mother died.

I go home and tell Angie, and, to my surprise, she seems really upset. 'What d'you go and do that for?' she wants to know. 'You've got *years* left.'

'I know,' I reassure her. 'But I just wanted it done. I've got to die one day, haven't I? And, if I've got to be buried alone, then I want to be with them. I can't think of anywhere I'd sooner be lying than at the side of your mum and dad.' I grin, trying to shake off her sad expression. 'Hey, it'll be just like when we used to be laid out at Rhyl, sunbathing,' I tell her. 'And I'll be able to have a good old chat with your dad.'

Angie smiles too, at last. Then she hugs me really tightly, not speaking.

But she doesn't really need to. For all my forced jollity about it all, the word 'alone' hangs too heavily in the air.

Chapter 13

Two days after Winnie's death we go back to the hospital to see the oncologist.

Angie's quiet, not herself, and I know she's missing her mum terribly. Every time I slip out of the house, to do my daily check on Herbert, or run an errand, I know she cries. I can tell by her bloodshot eyes. But she's like her dad, is Angie: she prefers to keep her grief hidden, to hold herself together, particularly for the children.

And now there's all this to deal with as well. Today's the day we are to hear the results of Angie's scan. And as we go to meet Lynne Handley of PALS – she's going to attend the meeting with us – I think we all know it's going to be bad news. I can tell even by the way Lynne looks so shocked when she sees us. I can see she's looking at Angie and noticing just how gaunt she is now. And it's not surprising. If she was struggling to eat before, she's finding it almost impossible right now. Grief has completely taken away her appetite.

Lynne knows nothing about Winnie dying, of course. 'How are you feeling?' she asks Angie, obviously noticing her pinched face. I tell her that Angie just lost her mum two days ago. 'Oh, Angie,' she cries. 'I'm so sorry. Look, would you like me to rearrange this appointment for another day?'

Angie shakes her head, and manages to find a small smile from somewhere. 'No, I'd rather just get it over and done with,' she says.

Even though we don't know what we're going to hear, the feeling of dread is still with me as the three of us file into the consulting room and take our seats. Angie's oncologist looks up briefly from her computer monitor, and explains that she's looking at the images right now. The atmosphere in the room is tense as she pulls them up on screen and studies them, and, when she turns to look at Angie, I can see she's really shocked, and also that she's about to deliver some bad news. And I'm right. Her face is a picture of sadness as she explains that there's been progression with Angie's cancer after all.

'I'm so sorry,' she says. 'But the cancer has spread now. There's progression in your lungs and bones, and there's also something new here.' She then explains that Angie now has a mass in her pelvis, which looks as if it's in one of her ovaries.

There's a silence in the room as we try to take this in, and I feel the tears once again prickling in my eyes. And then, after the consultant explains that it's now time to start Angie on some palliative chemotherapy, Angie does that incredible thing of making everyone else feel that bit better when, logically, it should be the other way around.

She smiles ruefully at the doctor and pats the top of her head. 'So I suppose I'll be losing this again?' she says.

The consultant nods sadly. 'I'm afraid so,' she confirms.

'Well this time,' Angie says firmly. '*I'll* be in charge. I'll have my sister-in-law shave the lot off as soon as I start.'

I glance at Lynne as Angie says this. Despite knowing how strong Angie is I think we're all shocked at how well she's taking everything, and once again I know that Angie's agreeing to this only for my and the children's sakes. After all, why would she want to put herself through chemo again? Why would anyone want to lose all her hair and feel constantly sick and ill? Not to mention losing her appetite, which Lynne also mentions to the doctor, who prescribes some supplements that will help build some strength up. And, now that Angie's teeth are gone, she's also able to be put on Zometa finally, to try to help contain the cancer in her bones. She's also got to have yet another scan, this time of her liver, in order to see what might be going on there.

We leave the office dazed, having so much to take in. But one thing sticks in my mind more than anything else. Our original appointment was booked for 14 November. We're only here now because I pushed to bring it forward. But, as the scans show there's been such progression with Angie's cancer, why didn't the hospital call us as soon as the results were through? Would they just have left it, growing unchecked, till then?

I say this to Lynne. Ask her what she thinks about it. 'Why didn't they call us in?' I ask her. 'If the scan showed the cancer had been progressing, why didn't they get in touch with us? If we hadn't asked them to move the appointment forward, we wouldn't be having it till the middle of November, would we?'

Lynne has no answer to this, obviously. How would she?

'I want to go back in,' I tell her. 'I want to go back in and ask the doctor.' So Lynne agrees to pop back in and see if the doctor will see me again. And she agrees, and I do. But she has no answer for me either.

'Mr Millthorpe,' she explains, 'I have only just received the scan reports myself, and I was as shocked as you were when I saw them.' And, since she hadn't thought there'd been any clinical signs of progression when she'd last seen Angie, she'd had no reason to think the scan would show that either. She explains that had she been sent the results a week previously, she would have brought the appointment forward herself.

'But if you're not happy with the situation, Mr Millthorpe,' she explains, 'then you can of course complain to the hospital.'

I tell her I might, much good it's going to do me. It's the here and now that we have to face, isn't it? That *Angie* has to face. When I get back outside, she's still looking as shell-shocked as when I left her, and, try as I might to calm down, because I know this isn't helping her, I'm finding it hard. I'm just too wound up.

'Are you okay?' asks Lynne. She can obviously see how agitated I am. 'Look, why don't you sit down for a few minutes?'

Angie does, lowering herself into a seat with a glazed expression on her face. But I don't do likewise. I can't. I'm too angry. It's all so frustrating, and I can't help wondering, what if? Perhaps it won't have made much difference to this vicious disease that's spreading inside her, but the not knowing really eats me up.

In the end, though, it's poor Angie who has to fight this particular battle, not me. She's the one who's got to take the horrible drugs, take the supplements, lose her hair, endure yet more scans and investigations, and get by without her teeth. It's such a lot of stuff to do, that it feels a little as if Angie were preparing to run a marathon, instead of what she's really doing: trying to hold off her death.

And in the midst of all this she has to bury her mother. Could life be any more unfair to her? I don't think so.

Ella's getting to the stage where she's needing a bit less sleep now, and with one thing and another – not least our trip to the hospital – she's had a longer nap than normal today, the result of which is that, at nine in the evening, she's wide awake.

As there's no point in trying to put her down till she's sleepier, we don't bother. She's never been a great one for going to sleep, Ella, and, given everything else that's been happening since just after she was born, we haven't the energy to come down on her hard. Instead, as she sleeps in our bedroom with us anyway, we've got into the habit of just letting her fall asleep on the sofa and taking her up when we go up ourselves. We've tried putting her to bed earlier, but she just screams the place down, waking all the other kids up in the process. And who in their right mind would want all those tears and upset at a time like this? She'll be asleep soon enough, and every day now is so precious.

And I can see that all too painfully clearly. Ella's sitting on the living room floor, playing with one of her dollies. It's her favourite one – the one she calls her princess doll, with a pink dress (Ella loves anything pink) and waist-length blonde hair. She's brushing it now, with a little pink hairbrush, chatting and giggling to herself as she does so, playing mummy to her, saying the same things Angie's always done with her.

The telly is on – some documentary programme about wildlife – but I know Angie's not really watching it. In fact, I can't help but notice how intently she's watching Ella.

'Oh, Mill,' she whispers, her cheeks glistening from all the tears that have been rolling silently down them. 'I so wanted to see all our children grow up.'

I put my arms around her and hold her tight and try to find the right words to say. But I can't find any, because there *are* none. We both know that Angie won't live to see them all grow up. I know we must be thankful that she's been able to be there for all of the three older boys' childhoods, but for the others there's so much still to come. And I can't even begin to let myself think about all the next steps in life – all those potential weddings and new babies. A whole clutch of new grandchildren to play with little Warren, perhaps. And, most upsetting of all, that chance to do as her mum did with her and go out shopping on a Saturday with her two daughters.

But none of it's to be. We can only think in terms of weeks and months. I pray so hard that, with the chemo she's going to be starting now, she'll still be with us to see Ella's fourth birthday. But beyond that I can't even bear to do the sums. All I know is that, if I could swap my life for hers, I gladly would. I would do it without a second thought. It's the unfairness of it all that hits me more than anything. It's just wrong. If one of us has to die, it should be me. After all, she's the one who carried each of them for nine months, and she's the one who has devoted every last bit of herself to raising them – and so well. Angie's whole reason for living has always been her family. Yes, I've been there too – of course I have – and, yes, I love them as much as she does, but she's their mummy. She's irreplaceable. Her children *need* her.

But we can't swap places, and it's constantly on my mind now that our children, one day soon, will be motherless. And, when that happens, I will have the terrifying, impossible-seeming task of trying to fill the void she'll leave behind. And it's obviously been on Angie's mind as well, because the following morning she surprises me with a question.

'Mill?' she goes, out of nowhere. 'What's Corey's birthday?'

It's midmorning, and I'm just back from doing all my errands: dropping the kids to school, popping into town to do some banking, and checking up on Herbert to see if he needs anything doing today. Now we're just sitting down for five minutes' peace and enjoying a cup of tea before I start preparing lunch, while Ella plays with her toys on the living room floor.

Our routine is so normal that you'd think life *was* normal, but then I know that's what Angie wants: to live life as we usually do, following the same routines and rituals we always did. Once we've had lunch and I've cleared the kitchen, it'll be time to collect the kids from school again, after which I'll have them change out of their uniforms, so they don't get them dirty, and then, while they're out playing with their friends and so on, I'll be making tea, followed by TV with us till around eight, then bath and bed. Same as every other weekday. Same as it will be for however many days we still have left. That's all she wants. To have those days keep happening.

I look at her now, confused. I'm not sure why she's asking. Corey's birthday isn't something she'd ever forget, after all.

'Thirteenth of December,' I say. 'At least, I think it is.'

Angie shakes her head. 'No, it isn't, Mill. It's the ninth. You're thinking of Connor. It's Connor who's birthday's on the thirteenth. Thirteenth of June, mind,' she adds. 'Not December.'

She smiles again, seeing that I'm getting the game she's playing here. 'Okay,' she says. 'Reece.'

'Seventeenth of April,' I say, and this time I do feel quite confident.

'No,' she says. 'Right month, wrong day again. It's Ryan whose birthday's on the seventeenth of April. Reece's is on the eleventh.' Angie puts her mug down on the coffee table. 'You've got to know the kids' birthdays, Mill. You've *got* to. What if you forget one of their birthdays? Can you imagine that? You mustn't *ever*. You've got to know all their birthdays by heart.'

She gets up off the sofa then, her tea only half drunk. 'You off somewhere?' I ask.

Angie shakes her head. 'I've got something for you,' she says, crossing the room to the fireplace. She reaches behind the clock on the mantelpiece and pulls something out. She brings it back and hands it to me. It's a notebook. An old school one of Connor's.

'Here,' she says. 'I've written them all down for you.'

I open the book. And there they are, the whole list of them, in date order, from Ryan's right through to Ella's.

Angie sits down beside me again, but not before tugging

her jeans up, because they no longer stay up by themselves. It's something she's been doing a lot these past weeks, and I'm not the only one who's noticed it, either. She just won't eat – not even the sort of stuff most people try *not* to. If I go to McDonald's to get the kids something, I always suggest she have a Big Mac – she used to love them – but she always shakes her head and says the same: 'Just get me a Happy Meal.' And I would be happy, too, if she'd just eat it when I do get it. It's so important that she build herself up.

'Have a good look at those dates and start learning them, okay?' she says now, 'Because I'm going to test you. I'm going to test you every day till you know them all by heart.'

I look at the list, already trying to memorise them, and there's something else there, too. Some other notes. What seems to be a short list of rules.

'What are these?' I ask, pointing to them. The first one reads, 'Plait the girls' hair or it splits'; the second says, 'Must do homework before bed.'

Just reading it chokes me up. When did she do this? The list of rules continues and extends to two pages – sixteen items, the last of which has been scribbled out.

'What's this one?' I ask her. 'This one you've changed your mind about?'

'It was going to be about making sure you get them off to bed,' she says. 'I was going to write that you need some time to relax after a hard day.' She grins at me. 'But then I realised you didn't really need that one.'

'Why?' I ask, perplexed.

'Because I know you. You'll be only too happy to get

them to bed, so you're not going to need me telling you, are you?'

She's right of course. As she is about the rest of them. It's nothing complicated. Nothing that I'd find difficult to achieve. Just a list of common-sense things I have to think of, day to day, such as remembering to take Ella for her meningitis booster, allowing the children only one hour a day of computer time, and checking their hair regularly for nits. And other things as well – wider things – such as vetting future boyfriends and girlfriends, making sure we all continue to go to Thornwick with the family every year. And obviously never, ever forgetting their birthdays.

It's really upsetting, visualising Angie sitting here thinking about this stuff, and by now I'm reading through a watery fog of tears.

'You don't need to worry,' I try to reassure her. 'We'll be fine. *They'll* be fine.'

Seeing how upset I am, she puts her arms around me. 'I know,' she says. 'I know, Mill. Come on, come here, you big softy.' Then she kisses me, and when she's done that her expression is firm. 'Have a good look at those dates, you hear? Any chance you get. Because I'm going to be testing you tomorrow, and the next day and the next one. I'm going to ask you every single day till you know all of them. By *heart*.'

I start that very morning. I check the list again, then put it back behind the clock and get some paper. Then start copying the dates out again, this time from memory. It feels a bit like I'm back in school, doing lines, or my times tables. And with the clock, just like in school, ticking onwards.

Chapter 14

Winnie's funeral is everything that we both know she would have wanted. It seems the sun has come out especially, to help us celebrate her life, and as we sing her favourite hymn, 'Jerusalem', I do feel a sense of celebration: as well as being a steadfast second mum to me all these years, she was also the mother who raised the woman I so love.

But her inspiring send-off is quickly followed with further trauma.

It's gone midnight by the time Ryan and Damon have gone home – a very long day. And by the time we get into bed I know Angie's shattered, so, when I can tell from her breathing that she's asleep, I'm glad. It takes me a while to drift off myself though: I can't help worrying about her – worrying that all this sadness is sapping her already fragile strength.

But it's going to prove to be a very short sleep in any case, as we're both woken again at around 2 a.m. by the sound of the phone ringing downstairs. It's always horrible hearing a phone ring in the middle of the night and I throw off the duvet with a knot in my stomach.

'It could be Dad, Mill,' Angie says anxiously, when I get out of bed to go and answer it.

It's not Herbert, though. It's my nephew Kane, my brother Terry's son. Terry's the brother who's married to Angie's eldest sister, Diane. We saw them only a few hours back, at the funeral.

'Uncle Ian?' he says. 'Can you come over to ours, quick? It's me dad – I think he's having a heart attack.'

I feel my stomach lurch. 'Okay, Kane,' I tell him. 'I'm on my way right now. Have you called an ambulance?'

He tells me he has, so I ring off and dash back upstairs to Angie, and once I've filled her in and she's reassured me she'll be fine, I head up to Terry and Diane's, some half a mile away.

By the time I arrive, Terry's already been put into the ambulance, lying on the stretcher with an oxygen mask on and wires attached everywhere. Diane's sitting beside him, looking grey. They're ready to get off now, so I tell them I'll follow along in the car, and all the way there I'm praying he'll pull through.

When we get to the hospital, the doctor puts Terry on an ECG machine and confirms it. It's a heart attack. Diane's terribly upset, and Terry is understandably frightened, and I spend an hour with them both just trying to help them stay positive and reassure Terry that the doctor says he's going to be okay.

It's 5 a.m. by the time I've dropped Diane off and returned home, and I try to slip back into bed quietly. Angie's dead to the world, Ella curled up alongside her, as ever, both their faces smooth and serene in sleep. Ella wakes, though – she's a light sleeper – which of course wakes Angie too. Though when I tell her about Terry's heart attack – which turned out to be quite a mild one – she seems pretty positive about his prospects. He'll be having a bypass, which should sort him out, and he'll be told to give up smoking and eat more healthily, but with no history of heart problems his prospects are good.

'He'll be fine,' Angie tells me, just before she drifts back off to sleep. She pats my arm. 'So don't you worry, Mill,' she says. And, as I drift off myself, I wonder about her confidence. Or is it just that she's no room left for further heartache?

There is one thing on Angie's mind, though, and I know what it is. It's the kids and what'll become of them when she's no longer there to mother them; and that list – the one she's written in the little notebook behind the clock on the mantelpiece.

So much has happened in the last week – Winnie's funeral and Terry's heart attack – that they have formed a kind of buffer against the stark news we were given so recently about her cancer: that it's progressed and is now growing elsewhere in her body. Which has perhaps been a blessing, in that it's forced us to concentrate on something else, but at the same time it's been a little like a cancer in itself – ever present and gradually eating away at us.

For Angie, I know it's been a point of no return. Yes, she'll start the chemo. But that's only because the scale of the enemy has grown so much, and Angie's now fighting something so much more powerful than herself. I know it's made her focus on the time when she won't be here to care for the children with a sense of urgency she didn't have before.

'It's all the little things,' she tells me, a couple of days later. 'It's all the tiny little things that are the biggest things, really. The things that make them feel the most secure.'

I know that sense of security is really on her mind now. We don't discuss it – it's too painful – but I suspect that, like me, she's thinking of the period of devastation our children have ahead of them, and what terrible times we are all going to have to live through when she goes. No amount of chicken curries or coconut buns or neatly ironed clothes – however vital – are going to get them through that on their own.

By now I *am* reasonably proficient at almost all the household chores, but, as with remembering their birthdays, there are still a zillion tiny things Angie does for the kids and, every time one occurs to her, she'll call and I'll come running. Just as she's doing now, while she's bathing Corey.

'You have to be careful not to get soap in his eyes,' she explains. She shows me how to hold my hand at the back of his neck and ask him to tip his head back when I'm rinsing the shampoo out. 'Otherwise he'll panic,' she explains. 'Won't you, pet?'

Another night she also shows me exactly how to soothe Ella after a nightmare. Ella still sleeps in our bedroom, as it's the only sensible place to put her, the two other bedrooms being already full to bursting. Reece and Connor share one room, and the younger three the other, on one of those double bunk beds, with a big bed on the bottom and a single one above. Jake and Corey sleep in the lower bed and Jade has the one on top, and, what with all their toys, there's hardly room to swing a cat as it is.

Which means Ella, who has a child-sized bed by now in our bedroom, more often than not clambers into bed with us. I watch and try to remember the precise way Angie scratches Ella's back, ever so gently, and am glad it's too dark for her to see the anguished expression on my face.

It's so hard to take everything in – correct birthdates included – but I know I have to do so, because the time will come (and please let it not come for a long time) when I will have to do all these little things, *every* time, myself.

But again I sense Angie has an even stronger sense of the clock ticking than I have. The following day – just a few days before she's due to start her chemo – it's the sort of autumn afternoon that's a real blessing: not too windy, dry and bright, with the sun low but warm still, and the younger kids, home from school now, are in the back garden, enjoying the chance to play out before it's dark.

Connor'll be back from his mate's soon, and Reece home from work, and it'll be time for me to make a start on tea. For the moment, though, we're enjoying a few minutes' peace and quiet, as they all run around and let off steam. Angie's standing in front of the fireplace mirror, brushing her hair, and I'm sitting in the armchair, reading the morning's newspaper.

We hear Ella crying before we see her. And it's a familiar

cry, too: she's either not got her way about something or taken a tumble in the garden. It turns out to be the latter: she comes into the room clutching her grazed knee theatrically, and, just as she's probably done scores of times before, runs straight across to her mum.

She's got her arms outstretched, waiting for Angie to pick her up and cuddle her, and I have no reason to think Angie will do anything other than what she always does. Despite her being so thin and frail now, and Ella having become so weighty, I still just expect her to scoop her up and make it better. In fact, I've got only half an eye on things and am still half reading the paper. It's an everyday kind of drama after all.

It's only when Angie speaks that I'm pulled up short.

'Ella, love, I'm busy. I've got things to do,' she tells her. And as I look up now, shocked, I see she's also pointing in my direction. 'Go to your dad,' she says to Ella. 'Let your dad nurse you. Go on.'

Ella looks up to her mum, then slowly lowers her outstretched arms. She's still sobbing, and I can see how bewildered she is. What's happening? Why doesn't her mummy pick her up and kiss her knee better?

Angie says nothing, though. Instead, she walks off at speed, into the kitchen. And, as she goes, I catch a glimpse of her face. She looks more distraught than I've seen her look in a long time. I throw the paper down, stretch my arms out and gather Ella into them, holding her close to stop her wriggling – she's still looking for Angie – going 'shh', and murmuring 'there, there' into her ear.

It's only a tiny graze – one more easily dealt with using a

kiss, rather than a plaster – and, as I can see Ella's tired now, I settle her on the sofa, scratching her back to soothe her, just as Angie's shown me. And within minutes she's happily snuggled down among the cushions, under a blanket, and dropping off to sleep.

When I walk into the kitchen, Angie's got her back to me. Her hair is shoulder-length again now and, despite how ill she is, it's still so thick and glossy, and I feel a pang, knowing how much she's dreading losing it all again. She's motionless, looking out into the garden, where the rest of the younger kids are still playing on the slide. She's also silent, but I already know she's been crying because I heard her when I was trying to settle Ella. I walk up behind her, put my arms round her and kiss her wet cheek.

'What's up, love?' I say, even though I already know the answer. 'Come on, tell me,' I urge, 'what's on your mind?'

She turns around then. 'Don't worry, Mill,' she says, wiping the tears from her face with the back of her hand, pulling herself together, trying to reassure me, as always. It feels all wrong, Angie always feeling she has to make me feel better when inside I know her own heart must be breaking. 'I just think it's better if the kids get used to running to you now, don't you?'

I shake my head automatically. It's almost an instinct. I can't stop it. 'Don't be talking like that, Angie,' I admonish her. 'As soon as you finish this lot of chemo, you'll be back in remission. You were stable for over twelve months after the last lot, remember. So who knows? You might have another full twelve months before you need to have more.'

Angie looks at me tenderly, but at the same time I think she's also slightly exasperated by what I'm saying. 'I don't think so,' she says quietly. 'Mill, this is it: it's spreading all over my body now.'

I shake my head. 'Angie, you'll be fine,' I say doggedly. But, though this time she doesn't contradict what I'm saying, I know it's only because she doesn't want to press what she believes to be true. So she'll go on now, I realise, with what she just did with Ella, even though I know how much it must be costing her, and putting the children's needs – their future sense of security – before her own. They need to come to me automatically when she's gone, every time, because, though I can't replace her, she's got the wisdom to know that if they can do that it will help them cope just that little more easily with having lost her.

Once again, I feel awed by my wife's incredible goodness, but at the same time it still feels like a punch in my solar plexus to know the pain this change in routine is going to put her through.

I try to think of something I can say to make it better. But, of course, there's nothing. So I just hold her and cry inside.

Chapter 15

As 14 October gets closer – the date Angie's chemo is to start – I am literally counting the days. And so is Angie, though, in her case, for different reasons. The day before – the kids in school, and Ella out with Natalie – I finish off preparing the veg for dinner, thinking Angie's in the living room watching telly, only to realise the telly's not even on.

I dry my hands, make us both coffees, thinking that perhaps she's just dozing, but when I go in there it's to find that she's not lying down: she's sitting in the armchair with her head bowed and her hand over her eyes.

'Love?' I say gently. 'I've made you a coffee.'

She doesn't answer, so I put the coffee down and kneel down in front of her. 'Angie?' I ask, touching the back of her hand. 'Are you okay?'

She puts her hand down and looks at me. Her face is wet, her eyes red. Still she doesn't speak. Just shakes her head.

'I can't bear it,' she says. 'Mill, I'm *dreading* it. And it's not even as if there's going to be anything at the end of it all, either.'

'Yes there *is*,' I insist. 'It's going to slow everything down. You'll be in remission again. You'll—'

'Yes,' she snaps back at me. 'But for how *long*? Months, if I'm lucky. It might only be weeks, mightn't it? Losing my hair again, being sick all the time . . . What's the *point*? How can I enjoy the time I have left with the kids feeling so terrible? How can it be worth it? The end result isn't going to change, is it? I'm still not going to be here to watch them grow up, am I? I'll still be *dead*.'

She bursts into tears then, big gulping tears. And I don't know what else to do but try to hold her. And after a while I go back to doing the only thing I can do: reminding her how precious to them even a few extra days will be. How it *is* worth it.

'God, Mill,' she says suddenly. 'Thank God you survived that brain haemorrhage. Can you imagine? What would happen to the kids now if you hadn't?'

I hold her tight and agree with her, but I don't thank God at all. If his plan had been to save me, to look after the kids after he decided to take Angie, then he got it wrong. He got it *so* wrong. It was *me* he should have taken.

The 14th of October arrives anyway, and Angie agrees she will start her chemotherapy, and I can't help but breathe a big sigh of relief. If she'd refused to take it, point blank, what could I do? But she hasn't, and, as soon as we get out of bed, I feel happier knowing the drugs will soon be coursing through her system, beating back the cancer that seems so intent on killing her. Though I know it's going to mean the start of another gruelling few weeks for her, it's such a comfort to know that it's actively under attack again. Even if they can't ultimately stop it growing, and we're going to lose her anyway, I so desperately want to keep her with us for those precious extra months, another Christmas, another spring, another round of birthdays, please God. *Please*, God – get at least this bit right.

I know Angie doesn't feel the same – I know she worries that I'm still hoping for a miracle – and, as we pull into a space at the hospital car park, I get the clearest signal possible that her mind is in a completely different place. I don't think she's been thinking about the precious few extra months the drugs might give her. The very opposite, in fact. She's been thinking about death.

She puts her hand on my left forearm as I switch off the ignition. 'Mill,' she says. 'Before we go in, I've got something I want to tell you.'

I turn to face her, trying to read her expression, wondering what it might be. Her expression is really serious and for a terrifying moment I think she's going to tell me she's found another lump.

But she doesn't. 'You know that grave you bought, Mill?' she says quietly.

The question's so unexpected that it takes me a couple of seconds to respond. 'Yes,' I say. 'What about it?'

'I've changed my mind,' she says. 'I don't want to be cremated any more. I want to be buried. I want you to put me in that grave you bought for yourself, Mill, so that I know one day we'll be together forever.'

I am so relieved I can hardly put it into words. I have been so dreading the thought of having to cremate Angie. This is exactly what I want: to have her there, waiting for me. It's not why I bought the plot, but now I am so incredibly glad I did – so incredibly glad that, when the time comes, I won't have to go through the horror of watching her coffin slide away into an incinerator.

'We'll always be together,' I tell her. 'Always, in my heart. I'm never going to love anyone but you, Angie. You know that.'

Angie shakes her head slightly. 'Mill, don't say that. You might meet someone else, and if you do, in the future, I want you to know that it's okay by me. You have your life to live, Mill, and I want you to be happy.'

Now it's my turn to shake my head. 'Angie, that's never going to happen,' I tell her. 'I love you. Always have and always will.'

'But in the future . . .'

I shake my head again. We've had the odd period of discord, like any other couple – usually when money was tight, the kids were small and both of us were stressed – but we'd always make up. We fitted. Right from the moment we started courting. I've loved Angie since I was fourteen years old and I'm not about to stop loving her. Not even when she's no longer with me. It doesn't work like that.

'Never going to happen,' I tell her, leaning across to kiss her. 'There's never going to be anyone in my life but you, I promise you.' I get out of the car and go round to open her door for her. 'Come on,' I say. 'No more talking like this.

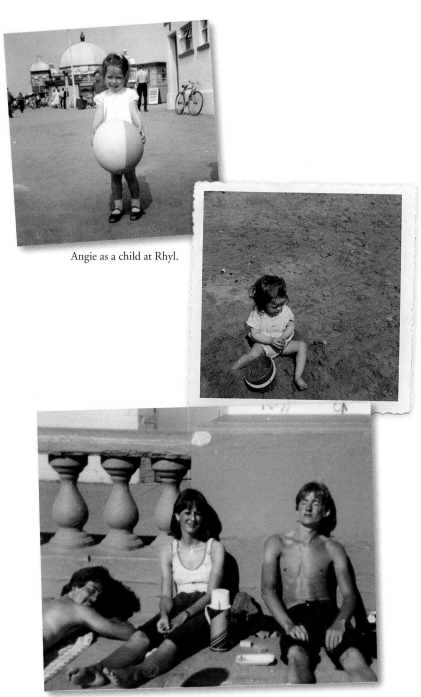

Angie as a child at Rhyl.

Me and Angie sunbathing with her brother Neil, back in Rhyl.

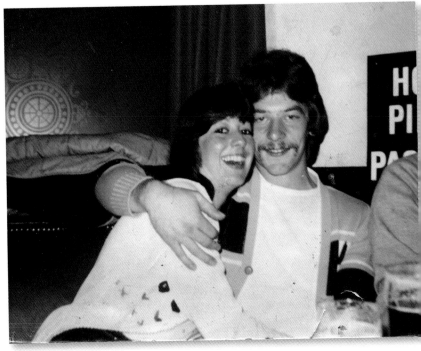

Angie and I on holiday – at Rhyl again – when we were both 18.

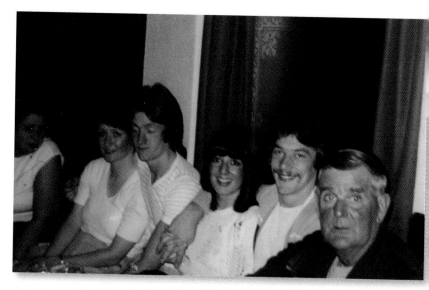

A night out with the family. From left to right: Angie's Mum Winnie, sister-in-law Diane with husband Neil, Angie, Me and Angie's dad Herbert.

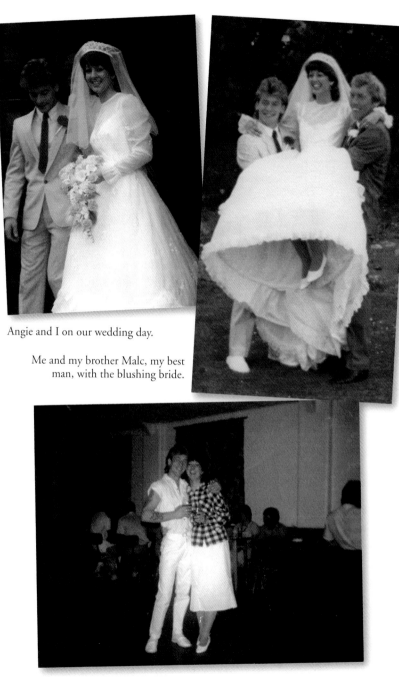

Angie and I on our wedding day.

Me and my brother Malc, my best man, with the blushing bride.

Wedding celebrations. I wore those trousers specifically to match Angie's shoes.

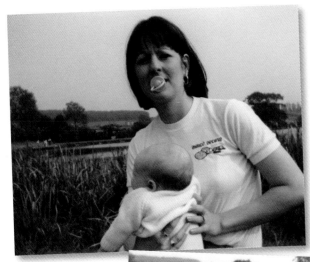

At the fishing lake in Grimethorpe Park. I expect Ryan is fishing for his dummy.

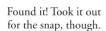

Found it! Took it out for the snap, though.

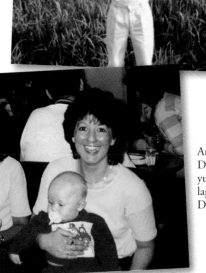

Angie and her sister Diane on holiday at – yup – Rhyl. On Angie's lap is Damon, and on Diane's, her son Kane.

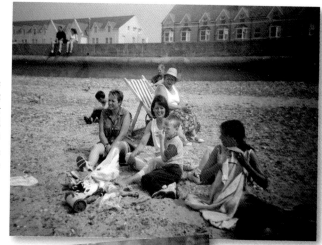

A picnic on the beach. Front, right to left: Angie's sister Diane, Angie and a friend. Behind: my second mum, Winnie, and Reece.

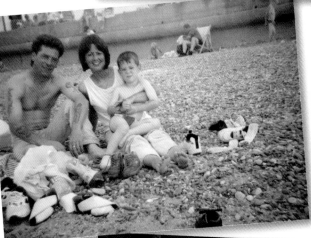

Me and Angie with Reece. And lots of footwear.

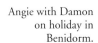

Angie with Damon on holiday in Benidorm.

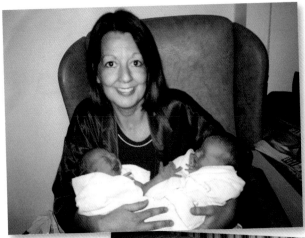

Angie in hospital after giving birth to Jake and Jade just hours before.

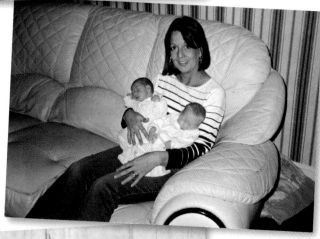

At home with the twins . . .

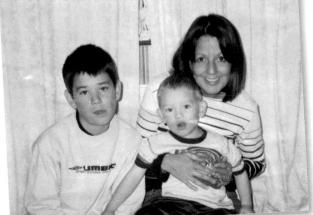

. . . and with Connor and Reece.

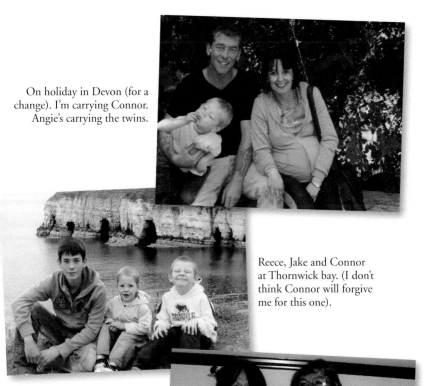

On holiday in Devon (for a change). I'm carrying Connor. Angie's carrying the twins.

Reece, Jake and Connor at Thornwick bay. (I don't think Connor will forgive me for this one).

Lynn's 50th. Angie is with my brother Malc's wife, Eileen, and is six months pregnant with Ella-Rose . . .

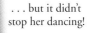

. . . but it didn't stop her dancing!

A night out with the family for Valentine's Day 2004. My brother Barry is in the front, then left to right: Barry's wife Lynn, my brothers Malc and Terry, Terry's wife Diane, me and Angie.

Champagne in the limo that same night with Barry and Lynn.

Angie, Ella and Corey, October 2009, at our beloved Thornwick Bay. This was taken just a year before Angie's death.

The list Angie wrote for me in an old school exercise book of Connor's.

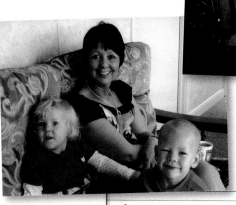

Ryan - 17-4-86
Damon - 29-3-89
Reece - 11-04-1991
Connor - 13-6-99
Jake - 21-11-02
Jade - 21-11-02
Corey - 9-12-05
Ella. - 22-6-07

① plait. gurls hair or it splits
② Must do homework. before bed.
③ Must be in 1 hour before dark.
④ Vet tv programmes.
⑤ Dont let them bite nails.
⑥ Vet boyfriends / gurl friends

⑦ Keep going to. Thornwick. with rest of family.
⑧ be strict with them.
⑨ Check their hair for nuts.
⑩ only one hour a day on computer.
⑪ Make sure ella. has her Meningitis boosters.
⑫ Dont have iron too hot for shirts.
⑬ Dont leave ella in bath alone.
⑭ Dont give them too many sweets.
⑮ Sun block on hot days.

You're not going anywhere – except up onto that ward and back into remission.'

Ward 24 is a bit like a drug itself. It's the ward where Angie had her chemo last time, so we know it well, and as soon as we arrive on it I feel the anguish of our conversation in the car ebb away a bit, to be replaced by a feeling of hope and positivity. I think Angie feels it too. There's just something about this ward that seems to lift everybody's spirits, and, though much of that's down to the sense of camaraderie that seems to exist here, the main factor is the incredible bunch of nurses. Everyone feels the same about the nurses on Ward 24: they are just fantastic and can't do enough for all their patients. They really are like angels on earth.

It's a different sort of ward from most. Though half of it's like a usual ward, with beds for inpatients – men and women – the other half's just for chemo. And on this side instead of bays it has lots of armchairs, because that's where the patients sit to have their drugs administered. They're given them via a drip, and the fluid takes about an hour to be infused, so it feels more like a social gathering than a medical environment – all the women (they all seem to be women) sitting around nattering to one another, telling stories and talking about how their cancer is affecting them and what stage of treatment they're at.

I stay with Angie for about fifteen minutes but, once she's been given a cup of tea and made friends with the woman sitting next to her, she suggests I pop along and see how my brother's doing.

Terry's still in Barnsley Hospital after his heart attack. He's in here recuperating and having regular blood tests in preparation for being transferred to Sheffield for his bypass operation.

He's looking well – very well, considering what he's just been through – and much more concerned about Angie than himself. And he's at pains to reassure me. 'She'll be fine, lad,' he tells me. 'You'll see. Once she's had her chemo, you wait – she'll be back to her old self again.' I hope he's right. I so want to believe him.

I certainly trust him. We're all very close, my brothers and sister and I, but Terry and I have always had this special bond. With his not having married when I was a child, and being the only driver in the house, he used to take me everywhere with him. He was a bit of a hero for me. 'Our Tekka' I used to call him. It seems incredible to me that he's sixty-five now. And that so much time has passed since I was a teenager courting Angie – not to mention that we ended up playing such a big part in finally finding him a wife.

But that's what happened. It was Angie's sister Diane's house that started it. She'd got divorced just before Angie and I met and, since she'd moved back to live with Winnie and Herbert temporarily, her house was sitting empty.

I remember it as if it were yesterday. It was a bitterly cold night in mid-December, and we were sitting, as we always were, freezing to bits on our step in the park. We didn't mind – it was the one place we could be alone together. But it was beginning to be a challenge, keeping warm. Not any more, though, it seemed, because that night Angie suddenly pulled a bunch of keys out of her coat pocket.

'*Ta-da!*' she sang, jangling them under my nose. 'Look what I've got!'

'What are those for?' I asked her.

'Our Diane's,' she said excitedly – she'd obviously been dying to tell me. 'They're the keys to her house. She's said we can go to hers instead of freezing to death out here every evening.'

I was open-mouthed. And, being a young man, instantly alert to the possibilities. I leapt up. 'Blimey! Why are we still sitting here, then?' I said.

It was a magical time. That first evening, Angie found some coal in the bunker and soon had a roaring fire going. And, now that we had a place – a warm and dry place – to do our courting, we felt the luckiest couple in the world.

It wasn't long, of course, till I realised there were even better possibilities. What would her dad think, I suggested a couple of months later, about our maybe staying nights there at the weekends? Angie was nervous. Yes, we were both working now, and had been together two and a half years, but Herbert was very strait-laced, and she was convinced he'd say no. But she was wrong. It was a big step, but he gave us his blessing, and from then it became our place – our little weekend love nest for two.

But all good things must come to an end, obviously – though in this case it was definitely for the greater good. Diane was round one day, a couple of years later, to see what might need doing, and, when she asked me if I knew anyone who might be able to do a bit of decorating for her, I suggested Terry – after all, he always did my mum and dad's decorating for them. 'He'll do it for you,' I told her. 'He's good at wallpapering, is Terry.'

Terry hadn't married yet, but that didn't mean he didn't have an eye out – and having seen Diane a couple of times, and knowing she was divorced now, he didn't hesitate to make the most of this unexpected opportunity. I should have known from his grin that he had plans other than just decorating, and, sure enough, he wasn't long into the job when Diane started popping round to help him. And it wasn't long after that that Angie and I realised we'd lost our love nest – it was more than wallpapering the pair of them were up to.

So now everyone was happy. They were married that same December.

However, my more positive mood, both from being on the ward and from seeing Terry, doesn't seem to extend beyond the hospital. And, when we emerge back into the car park, and I can see how withdrawn Angie is, I'm catapulted back into reality with a real jolt. She's so quiet – so not her usual, positive, can-do self – and I wonder if she's heard some bad news about another patient, or maybe it's just hit her what a gruelling few weeks she has ahead.

We get into the car and begin the drive home and the atmosphere feels really gloomy. It's that kind of day, as well, the sky a dirty grey, the dead leaves piling up in soggy heaps everywhere. And it's not even as if we could just concentrate on looking forward to Christmas: with the chemo under way,

I doubt Angie can even bear to think of Christmas, because, with the drugs knocking her sideways and her being sick all the time, it'll be such a struggle to do it all, however much she'll want to spoil the children.

Not for the first time, I can understand why some people choose not to go through with chemo. Yes, Angie coped reasonably well with it before – in the end, at least – but things are different now: she's so much weaker. It'll be a real slog for her, and I really wish I could just take the drugs for her.

I look across at her as we drive. She's just sitting there, saying nothing. She's got her hands in her lap and she's twiddling her rings round and round her finger. They feel like a part of her, Angie's rings, and she's never taken them off. She took off her engagement ring only once: to allow me to put the wedding ring on her finger. They have stayed there, in place, ever since. Her eternity ring, which is also gold, with diamonds and rubies, was something I bought for her in Rhyl. It was during a night out at the Victory Club there that I gave it to her. I told her I fancied a quick walk along the prom together, and, once we were out there on our own, I produced it with a flourish, slipping it over her finger to join the other two.

I look at her profile now and I wonder what she's thinking. I don't ask her, though. Somehow I don't think probing her thoughts is what she wants. Instead I wait till I find a suitable place to pull over. I can't drive any more, anyway. My heart's too full for me to be able to concentrate.

I pull in on the stretch of road that forms a bypass between Cudworth and Shafton. The road is flanked by open fields in which horses are grazing, and one or two look up curiously as I swing the car in and come to a stop.

'What you doing, Mill?' Angie asks, confused, as I pull up the handbrake.

'I've just been thinking,' I tell her. 'Your last dose of chemo is in March, right? So here's the plan. Soon as we get home, I'm going to get on the Internet, and I'm going to book us into the St George's Hotel again. Would you like that? For straight after you finish chemo. So we can celebrate. And for a whole week this time. What d'you think?'

Her face brightens immediately. 'Oh, Mill, I'd love that,' she says. And, though I know it's just my clumsy male way of trying to find a solution when there isn't one, the fact that she grabs for it anyway – grabs it like a lifebelt – cheers me up no end. I think we both need to see something happier on the horizon. 'Oh, Mill,' she says again. 'I would *really* love that.'

Her face opens out into a smile then, as something else occurs to her. 'Better borrow our Neil's satnav again, then,' she jokes. 'Or maybe even splash out and get our own one.' Then she grins, and it's like the sun coming out, even if it is only inside the car. 'Mind you, I missed visiting Cheadle last time,' she muses. Then she laughs. A proper Angie laugh. 'Not really!'

It's not much – just a plan to go on a break the following spring. But it's something to aim for, at least. Something to look forward to. Something to help us both believe that, since we've made plans, death can clear off for a bit. She's bloody well going to live to see them happen.

Chapter 16

It's just as well Angie's taught me so thoroughly, because I'm becoming paranoid about her not getting enough rest now she's back on chemo. She might feel she's doing okay, but it'll knock her for six in no time, and I'm determined to make sure she's as strong as she can be. She's always so reluctant to take a nap, and I understand that: she can hear the clock ticking; it must be like a drum in her head. But I have to be firm. She's so skinny and so weak – she just doesn't see it. And she needs her strength more than ever; needs to muster whatever reserves she can. It's as though we were in two opposing teams, death and I, and I've got the upper hand now – just as long as the chemo can do what it needs to, and give Angie a little extra time. And, in truth, I need to do it, anyway, just to prove to her I can. I need to do the lion's share of everything: run the house, manage the kids. I need her to know I won't crack up and let her down. I need to know it for myself as well – because the enormity of the responsibility I have ahead of me is kicking in now. I have eight kids, the youngest six of them still under my roof. All those young lives about to be dependent on me utterly.

The 18th of October is a school day, a Monday, after what's been a really nice, and unremarkable, weekend. And one in which life really seemed to feel reasonably positive. That first dose of chemo is such a weight off my shoulders – I don't think I realised just how big a boulder had been sitting there till last Thursday's session lifted it from me.

But even that makes me feel guilty, because I know she's the one who now has to endure it. I just pray it won't hit her so badly that she won't want to carry on.

On the Saturday we stayed in and had a takeaway, just as we always do, and sat down all together, to watch *The X Factor*. Angie loves *The X Factor* and this year she's really keen on Storm Lee, whom she has been following since the auditions. The kids are all mad about One Direction, but for Angie Storm's the best of the bunch. 'He'll walk it,' she kept saying. 'He's just got such a wonderful voice. He's going to make the finals for definite.'

The finals happen close to Christmas, but my mood was still so positive. Now Angie was back on chemo, I felt confident she'd be seeing the New Year. But perhaps she didn't feel as confident as I did – I don't know. Or perhaps she was better than I was at dealing with the reality. While I coped with the future by pushing it to the back of my mind, Angie always seemed to want to do the opposite.

We'd just finished our takeaway, and were on the sofa, watching the final bit of *The X Factor* when Ella, who'd fallen asleep right there on the carpet, woke up crying, and immediately grizzled at Angie to be picked up. It was such an automatic thing and Angie's response was automatic now, as well.

'Go to your dad, Ella,' she said quietly. 'Go on – he'll nurse you.'

I held my arms out. 'Come here, love,' I said. 'Come on. Let me nurse you.' But she still toddled to Angie, holding her own arms out, trying to climb onto her mum's lap.

'Aw,' said Angie. 'Poor Dad! I bet he thinks you don't love him now! *Poor* Dad!' She made a big show, then, of putting her head on my shoulder and snuggling up to me. '*Poor* Dad!' she said again. 'Come on, Dad, you can nurse me instead.'

It worked like magic. Ella immediately climbed up onto my lap and cuddled me, while Angie looked up at me and gave me this satisfied little smile. Then it was Corey's turn. Turning round to see me cuddling both Angie and Ella, he clambered up as well, wanting a cuddle too. And it was lovely, the four of us there, all cuddled up on the sofa together. Except that I couldn't quite shake off the horrible feeling of why what had just happened *had* to happen.

But I had to, and I did, and the rest of the weekend was lovely. Sunday was dry, so, after popping to see Herbert and having a lunch of roast beef, we took the younger kids to Hemsworth Water Park. It's only a couple of miles away from us, and has a lake with a sandy beach and a big children's play park that the kids love. And, after they'd worn themselves out, we fed the ducks with stale bread we'd saved specially for the purpose, because Angie hates wasting food when there's some poor hungry bird that can make use of it.

Sunday night came around then, and Storm didn't make it through to the next round of *The X Factor*. Didn't even make the sing-off, unfortunately. But One Direction are still in, which makes the kids happy, Jade particularly. She adores them. Angie and I aren't so sure. Five-minute wonders? We shall see.

The start of a school day is the usual military exercise. And, because I need Angie to really keep her strength up now she's back on chemotherapy, I am really firm about her not doing *anything* that might tire her. I sort the children out for school downstairs while she has a lie-in, little Ella tucked up and fast asleep beside her. I get the rest up at 7.30 and make them breakfast while they watch cartoons on the telly. Then, once they've all had their cereal at the kitchen table, I deal with Corey and help Jade and Jake, up in the bathroom, while Connor gets himself dressed and organised.

Reece works just down the road from us, but he's long gone by this time. He's generally up before all of us, usually at 6.30, and heading off to work just before the rest of us are downstairs. Then it's hair – I'm getting better now, and keen to keep practising, so I quickly do Jade's for her in front of the fireplace. It's not perfect (we both know that) but it's not terrible either and, bless her, she pronounces it just fine.

And that's us all done and set to go. Just time for a quick dash upstairs to give Angie a kiss, then they all thunder back down again, ready.

'See you later, Mummy!' they all trill as they clatter out. Because why on earth would any of them think they wouldn't?

*

The kids delivered to school, I pop in to see Herbert. He tells me he's okay, just as he tells me every day, but he's quiet, and when I press him he admits he's not planning on making himself dinner.

'You've got to eat something,' I tell him. 'I'll fetch something for you.'

But he shakes his head. 'Mill, there's no need,' he says.

'Yes, there is,' I say. 'I'll bring you a piece of fish round from the fish-and-chip shop.'

And I think he realises that I'm not taking no for an answer. 'Twelve o'clock or so,' I tell him. Then I hurry home.

When I get back I'm surprised to see Angie's already up and about. She's already washed and dressed too. Not only that: she's also busy cleaning the kitchen worktop, while Ella looks on from her high chair.

I put down my car keys and give Angie a stern look. 'Hey,' I say. 'What do you think you're doing? You're supposed to be resting!'

She laughs her usual laugh. 'Oh, Mill,' she says. 'I'm *fine*.'

Fine? No, she's not. That's such an overused word. *I* overuse it. She's not fine at all: she's dying. But, even though she's so frail and skinny now, her smile still lights up the room. How can that be? How can someone so ill still manage to look so radiant? And so determined? Which she does look. She won't have it.

'Look,' she says, doing a little twirl as if to prove it. 'I've already cleaned the kitchen floor as well.'

And it's perhaps that – that little dance she does in the middle of the kitchen – that makes everything that happens subsequently so shocking.

'Well, you're not doing any more,' I tell her, holding my hand out for the cloth and spray bottle of kitchen cleaner she's holding. 'You're going to put your feet up and have a cuppa and get some *rest*.'

Angie doesn't argue – I think she knows that I'll not be swayed on this – so, instead, she goes into the lounge with Ella and puts the telly on while I make tea.

'So how's me dad?' she wants to know, once we're both on the sofa and Ella's playing with her dolls on the floor. I tell her he's quiet but that he's had his breakfast and that I'm going to get some lunch for him.

She nods. 'He'll be fine. He just gets on with it, doesn't he?'

'I know,' I say. 'But I still worry about him. He's really missing Winnie. And we don't see what he's like behind closed doors.'

Angie pats my arm. 'He'll be fine, Mill. We'll all get him through this.'

And it's just when I'm thinking how typical of Angie that is – to be so caring when she's going through so much herself – that I realise she's lapsed into silence.

'You okay?' I say, turning to look at her.

She shakes her head slightly. 'Mill,' she says, putting her tea down, 'I don't feel well.'

I look at her properly now. Her skin suddenly looks different: pale and clammy.

I put down my own tea and go to fetch a pillow to support her, fluffing it up at the end of the sofa so she can lie down for a bit.

'You rest there for a while,' I tell her. 'See, I told you not to overdo it. You just rest. It's probably just the chemo kicking in.'

She does as I suggest but she still doesn't feel any better. 'I feel sick, Mill,' she tells me, swallowing. 'I feel *really* sick.'

She tries to get up then, but before she can get on her feet she vomits – a rush of dark brown, all over the cream leather sofa.

Telling Ella to come upstairs with us, I half help, half carry Angie up the stairs to the bathroom, where I strip her of her soiled clothes and wash and change her.

And to my relief, she says she doesn't feel so sick any more. Though now she has a pain in her left side. 'Down here,' she says, pointing to the lower left of her stomach.

'Come on,' I say, 'let's get you back down on the sofa till you feel better.' But she doesn't. Another half-hour passes and she continues to feel worse, so I carry her upstairs to bed instead.

At noon, I decide to get the doctor. I'm anxious that he examine her and see what might be causing it. It might be the chemotherapy poisoning her, after all. I call my brother Glenn then, and ask him if he'll get Herbert's promised fish for him. 'But just tell him Angie's feeling a bit poorly,' I tell Glenn. After what he's been through already, I don't want him worrying unnecessarily. Glenn's also going to pick Corey up from nursery for me, then come and mind Ella while I drive to the GP's. I'm so grateful. I honestly don't know what I'd do without him.

By now I'm getting anxious that Angie's had some terrible reaction to the chemo, and, when I return from the surgery and see Malc and Eileen pulling up at their house, I tell them what's happening. They drop what they're doing and say they'll pop over too, so they can give her a bit of extra support.

The doctor, a young Asian woman with long black hair tied in a ponytail, arrives around half an hour later. But, when I ask her about the chemo, she says she feels it's probably not that. She takes a look at Angie and gives her something to help ease the pain, and tells us it's too soon for it to be likely to be related to her chemotherapy.

'We need to be sure, of course,' she says, 'but I doubt it. It's more likely to be related to the mass on your ovary,' she says to Angie. 'But, either way, we need to get you to hospital.'

She calls the hospital herself, but, because it's not strictly an emergency, tells me it'll be quicker for me to drive Angie there than to call an ambulance.

We arrive at Barnsley Hospital at around 2.20 and, by now, I'm pleased to see that Angie has some of her colour back, and tells me she's beginning to feel a little better. In fact, she starts getting out of the car almost as soon as I park.

'What are you *doing*?' I want to know, coming round to her side of the car.

She smiles. 'What do you think? We're going into the hospital, aren't we?'

'Yes,' I say. 'But you stay right there while I go and get you a wheelchair.'

Angie laughs out loud at this. 'Get out of here, stupid!' she says. 'I don't need a wheelchair. I can walk!'

'Yes, but you're *not* walking,' I say firmly. 'Besides, if I put you in a wheelchair, you can hold the bowl on your lap, which means that if you're sick again it won't go all over the hospital floor.'

She shakes her head and flaps a hand at my undeniable logic. 'Oh, go *on*, then. If it makes you feel better, Mill.'

She's still grinning at me as she climbs into it.

We've been told to go straight to Ward 18 when we arrive, and, once we're there and a nurse shows Angie to a bed, the doctor asks me to tell him about her recent treatment. 'Do you know what medication Angie's currently on?' he asks me. I tell him I don't – there's just so much of it – but that I've brought everything along with me, and he tells me that, while I go back out to the car to fetch it, he'll go and take a look at her notes and the latest scan.

He's still doing so when I return to Angie's bedside. Once he's done, he comes and tells us that, judging from her scan, the GP's correct: the pain is in all likelihood coming from the mass on her ovary.

Angie's in pain again, the painkillers the GP gave her having worn off now, and the nurse gives her a new dose of pain relief.

'Just press the button,' she says, pointing to it, 'if the pain's still there after fifteen minutes, and I'll come back and give you another dose.'

'Can't I go home with my husband?' Angie asks her. 'The pain's not too bad now.'

The nurse shakes her head. 'No, I'm sorry. You'll have to stop here tonight so we can get your pain under control and keep you under observation.'

Angie's really upset about this unexpected development. 'But I want to go home,' she says. 'I can't be stuck in here. I need to be home for the children.'

It's not an option today, and, much as I'd like to take her home with me, I can see she's really struggling to put a brave face on how she's feeling. And I agree with the doctor: it would be mad to take her home when she's in this amount of pain. And they may also be able to do something to help her.

She must be in a lot of pain because they have to come and give her more relief not long later – so much so that, by around four, she's fast asleep. I stay for another half-hour or so, watching her sleeping, then decide to head back home for a bit. The kids will be home from school now – Reece home from work, as well, probably – and I'll need to give them all their tea. I kiss her forehead and tell her I'll be back around 6.30.

When I get home, Damon and Natalie are already there: Damon to come back with me to visit his mum, along with Reece, and Natalie, bless her, to help mind the little ones. I call Ryan, too, and suggest we pick him up on the way.

If the little ones are aware of the drama unfolding around them, they at least *seem* oblivious. With the family all being so close, they're used to lots of comings and goings. Their main need right now is for food. Only once I'm finished with the cooking does Corey seem confused.

'Where's Mummy?' he wants to know, as I dish up their food: fish fingers, peas and chips, what they all asked for.

'She's just got a bad tummy ache, that's all,' I explain. 'So she's going to sleep in the hospital tonight and will be back home tomorrow.'

More interested in the plates set in front of them now, the younger children seem to readily accept this. All bar Connor, I realise, who has his head down and is silent. I worry that he understands more than I'd like to think. Reece and I exchange looks. I've already told him, while he was upstairs in the bathroom, having his wash. I can tell he's as strung out as I am.

But, for all my anxiety about Angie being in pain, I've told the little ones nothing that isn't true in saying that Mummy will be home again tomorrow. Because not once – not even for a fraction of a second – does it occur to me that she might not.

Chapter 17

While the children eat their tea, I remain positive. After all, as the oncologist said before, Angie responds really well to chemotherapy, and we've been told that, when someone responds as well as Angie has done so far, there are so many options still open to us. So we'll get past this blip, I think, and, once the chemo starts working, I feel confident we'll have Angie well again. Only for a bit – I'm not stupid – but every bit is so precious.

I return to the hospital with the two oldest boys at 6.30, just as I've promised, having driven and picked up Ryan on the way. Both, by now, are settled and living with their respective girlfriends and working hard for a local firm, installing kitchens. They're grown men now – Damon is a father himself, of course. But they are still our babies, and always will be, and I have this huge sense of anguish about how much losing their mum is going to hurt them.

But that's for another day. She can get over this, I know she can. They'll find some way to deal with whatever it is that's hurting her. And soon the chemo will start to shrink the cancer again anyway. Even so, I keep getting knocked for six, ambushed by my feelings. As we pull into the hospital car park I stop to let a young couple cross the service road. They're pushing a baby in a pram, and could just as easily be Damon and Natalie, and it suddenly hits me really hard that, whatever happens at the hospital tonight and tomorrow, this is a one-way journey we're going on, and that Angie's not going to be around to watch her little grandson grow up. Won't be there for when our other kids have children.

But right now my one concern is that we get over this hiccup, get Angie home again, and well again, and fast. She's still dozy when the boys and I arrive back in her room up on the ward, and for the first fifteen minutes or so the three of us simply sit around her bed.

After a while, though, she finally opens her heavy eyelids and smiles a little to find us back with her.

'Has the pain gone now, Angie?' I ask, squeezing her hand.

Angie shakes her head slightly, and pulls the same face I saw earlier. 'No,' she says. 'It's not, Mill.' She gestures to her lower stomach again. 'It's still there.'

'Okay, love,' I say, rising. 'I'll go and fetch a nurse for you.' I then go off outside to find one to see if they can do something.

The nurse returns with me and asks Angie the same thing that I did, and Angie explains that it feels a bit like a labour pain.

I smile at Angie. 'And you know what they feel like,' I say. 'Don't you, love?' Then I turn to the nurse. 'She's had eight children,' I explain.

The nurse smiles at the boys, and tells Angie she'll sort her pain out for her, and when she returns a few minutes later, she has a syringe of something with her – a clear liquid, which she squirts into Angie's mouth.

It has the desired effect. Soon Angie's no longer wincing from the pain and is back breathing steadily, and very soon she seems to be fast asleep. It's a quarter to eight now. Almost the end of visiting time.

'I think we might as well head home again,' I tell the boys. 'Don't you? Get some dinner while Mum gets some rest.'

Just as we're leaving a male nurse comes in to check on Angie. 'How's my wife doing?' I ask him, as he checks her chart.

'Okay,' he says. 'We'll just make sure we keep her pain under control, and in the morning she'll be transferred over to a Macmillan nurse. They'll take good care of her.'

He smiles and I feel reassured that all's well. I lean down, kiss Angie's cheek and we head for home.

By the time we've dropped Ryan off and got back to ours, Damon and I are both starving. Reece and the girls have eaten, but neither of us has yet, so I open the fridge to see what's in there and decide to cook us both a full English.

'How's Mam?' Reece asks, and I can see he's looking worried, so I hurry to reassure him she's okay. 'Not in pain now,' I tell him. 'But she's been knocked out by the drugs. Fast asleep now. Best thing for her.'

Which is exactly what I'm thinking – that Angie's in the best place – so when I hear the house phone ring, as I'm finishing off the cooking, I just assume it's another family member wanting to hear how she is. But, when Reece appears in the kitchen with the phone in his hand, I can tell right away that it's not. He holds it out for me to take.

'Dad, it's for you,' he says. 'It's the hospital.'

I take it from him, put it to my ear and say hello. It's a woman's voice. She asks if I'm Mr Millthorpe and when I tell her I am she introduces herself as one of the nurses who are now looking after Angie. I feel a stab of worry. Why would they call me at this time in the evening? Is she in pain again? Has she been asking for me, maybe?

I have no idea what it might be, but, if she needs me there to support her, food can wait. However, it's worse than I could possibly imagine. 'Mr Millthorpe,' the nurse says slowly, 'you came to visit your wife earlier, didn't you?'

'Yes, I did,' I confirm. 'Is she okay?'

'I'm afraid she's taken a turn for the worse. Just after you left the hospital, unfortunately. I think it would be best if you came back as soon as you can,' she says. Then there's a pause. 'And bring your family, as well.'

I stand and stare at Reece, poleaxed. I can't stop looking at him, and I can see my own fear reflected so clearly on his stricken face. And then I start shaking, as the nurse's words press ever more insistently, smothering me. 'Okay,' I manage to get out. 'Okay. I'm on my way.'

It's the words. It's the memory of that phone call only weeks back. The same tone, the same words. *Come back. Bring your family.* The same words they used to tell us Winnie was going to die soon. Taken a turn for the worse. Come back. Bring your family. *Say goodbye.*

I feel a kind of rage begin to rise up inside me. It explodes from my mouth. 'Oh, God! I'm going to lose her! *I'm going to lose her!*' And without even realising what I'm doing I hurl the phone onto the kitchen floor. It seems to explode into a billion pieces, and, as Reece darts to retrieve them, I start slamming my fists as hard as I can down on the kitchen worktop, till my legs refuse to support me any longer and I crumple into a heap on the kitchen floor.

Damon rushes in then, Natalie close behind him, and together with Reece they manage to scrape me up off the floor. The kids are clamouring behind as well now – I catch a glimpse of their terrified faces – and Sophie and Nat rush to bundle them back into the living room. 'Come on,' Reece is saying to me, his voice cutting through the fog of terror. 'Dad, *c'mon*,' Damon adds. 'Let's get you to the hospital.' Together, they haul me out to Damon's car.

On the way, I gather enough presence of mind to think rationally, and have Reece call Angie's brother Neil, so he can tell everyone what's happening. 'Not Herbert, though,' I tell him. 'I can't put Herbert through this.' He's only just buried his wife. And he's so old now. Having to watch his daughter die would just be too much for him.

I feel the thoughts clamouring in my head. Because that's what's going to happen. That's why they want us there now. They need us to come because *Angie's going to die.*

Reece also calls Ryan, who is waiting at his front gate as we pull up, and the three boys and I arrive at the hospital around ten. We're met by a nurse, but shown up to a different ward now, because they've moved Angie to a private room. We can't go in straightaway, though. Instead, we're taken to a small waiting room.

'The doctor will come and talk to you in here,' she explains. 'He won't be long.'

We nod mutely. None of us know what to say. By now, the rest of the family start arriving as well: Malc and Eileen, my sister Karen, Neil and Diane, Angie's brother Des, her sister Wendy, and then Terry's Diane, together with her grown-up son, Jonathan, whom she had with her first husband. But not Terry himself, because he's still in hospital in Sheffield recovering from his recent bypass.

We all find seats and I glance around me. Everyone's ashen. Terrified. Teetering on the edge of tears. It doesn't matter that everyone always knew this day was coming. No one is ready. It's too soon. We're all in shock.

The on-call doctor, a woman whom we've not dealt with before, comes in and shuts the door quietly. She stands in front of us all but her eyes are fixed on me.

'Just after you left, your wife vomited a small amount of blood, Mr Millthorpe, and shortly after that – at nine p.m. – she had a cardiac arrest. We did manage to get her back,' she goes on, 'but we think she may have had a stress-related ulcer burst. Your wife is very ill, Mr Millthorpe,' she adds quietly, looking directly at me, 'and we don't think she's likely to survive the night.'

I break down again, and Karen and the boys and I cling together. I simply can't process this. None of us can. We're all sobbing as the consultant continues with what she needs to say. 'If she does survive the night,' she says, 'then in the morning we can put a camera down to find out what's going on, obviously ...' She stops then, because there's nothing more to say.

The nurse touches my shoulder. 'Come on, Mr Millthorpe,' she says. 'Follow me. I'll take you down to your wife so you can have a few minutes alone with her, and then the rest of the family can come in a few at a time. We can't have everyone in at once, because the nurses need to keep coming in to see to her.'

I can barely take any of this in. I follow her in a trance, stumbling, hardly able to function, while the rest of the family support the boys. I'm racked with pain now. How can this have happened so suddenly? How could she have been laughing in the kitchen only this morning and be suddenly so close to death? *How?*

I pray so hard. I've barely set foot in a church since my marriage, but I pray anyway – I have no idea what else to do. And when I see Angie lying there, so still and frail, with an oxygen mask over her face, all I can do for a few seconds is stand there and cry while a knife tears and slashes inside my stomach.

I climb up on the bed then and lie down beside her, with my arm around her, as if God won't take her if I hang onto her, if he can see she belongs here still, if he can just tell how much we all still need her. 'Please Angie,' I whisper to her, 'don't go. Please hold on. Don't leave me. Please God, don't take her, she means the world to us.'

The night inches by – I am clinging onto the idea of 'the morning' like a talisman – and we all sit and will her on, stroking her hair, holding her hand, and every one of us fixated on her breathing. She takes a breath, breathes it out, then there's this terrible long pause, which has all of us holding our breath as well.

By 2 a.m., though, there's a change, and all of us can see it. Bit by bit, her breathing has become steadier and more regular, and those scary pauses seem to have gone away. We're all allowing ourselves to smile now. Perhaps she's turned a corner, weathered the storm after all. I even find myself looking at Neil and Diane and, despite my tears, smiling.

'She's going to open her eyes in a minute,' I say, 'and tell us we're all crackers. "Warra all you lot doing crying at the side of my bed? Get yer sens home! I'm *fine*! Just having the lot of you on, that's all!"'

And, even though she doesn't, we are all feeling so much better. The tension's eased and the fear has been lifted from our shoulders. We're none of us going home, though: we need to see her through till dawn, when I'm beginning to believe she'll wake up again and grin at me. 'Mill,' she'll say, 'stop worrying! I'm *fine*!'

But for now she's sleeping peacefully, and I'm grateful. And also stiff, because I've not left Angie's bedside for five hours. So, when Angie's sister Diane says she wants to pop outside for a cigarette, I tell her I'll come down and keep her company. She doesn't want to go by herself because it's the middle of the night.

'You'll keep an eye on her?' I say to Malc. 'We won't be five minutes.'

Malc nods. 'You go on, lad,' he says. 'Go and get some air.'

We make our way down in the lift, both agreeing how much better Angie's breathing seems now. I even manage to make a joke. 'You know what?' I say, as the lift deposits us back down on the ground floor. 'I'm going to give her a right ticking off in the morning, having us all here at this time of night!'

The air outside is cold and, after so long in the warmth of the hospital, it hits me like a slap. But it's good to breathe it in, knowing Angie's so much more settled. I look up at the sky and will it to lighten. The dawn can't come quickly enough now.

But it seems there is to be none. Not for Angie. Because no sooner are we out there – can't be more than a minute – than the eerie small-hours silence is shattered by the hiss of an electronic door. I turn around to see, and gasp to recognise the figure of my nephew Jonathan, thundering out of the hospital entrance. 'Mill,' he says, panting. 'You've got to come in and sit down.'

I know straightaway. I know as soon as I see Jonathan's expression. I don't sit down. I dodge past him, take the lift back up to Angie's ward and run back down the corridors to Angie's room, the tears streaming down my face. '*No!*' I cry. '*No!*'

I get back to the ward to see everyone crammed outside Angie's room, see everyone crying, their shoulders shaking, hear the wretched sound of sobs. They make way for me, and, just as I get to where the door is, I see my boys, all there together, hugging. Reece is looking out for me, his face streaked and puffy. 'I think she was waiting,' he whispers in my ear as we cling together. 'Waiting for you to leave so you wouldn't have to see her go, Dad.'

Chapter 18

The world I gaze out on now, from the window of my brother Malc's car, feels strange, new and very, very frightening. It's not even six yet, and the sky is fully dark, with no hint of the dawn I prayed so hard Angie would live to see. I don't want to see it now, either.

But it's a new day, even so. And a very different one. It's the day I've known was coming for a very long time now – the first day of my life, since I was a fourteen-year-old lad, without the woman I love by my side. I catch my breath. I can't believe how scared and alone I feel.

I couldn't stay there in the hospital. I couldn't bear to.

As I walked into the little room, and saw Malc and Diane clung together crying, I felt physically sick, I was so frightened. I was frightened about what I was about to have to deal with, frightened about how I'd react when I saw Angie lying there, frightened about whether I'd be able to hold myself together in front of everyone.

As soon as I laid eyes on her I could see there was no longer breath in her body. I could see she'd gone, but I rushed to her side anyway. I pulled her close to me, wrapped her in my arms and sobbed into her hair. The hair she wouldn't lose now, after all. 'Don't leave me, Angie,' I whispered. 'Please don't leave me. How will I tell the kids? How will I go on?'

But as I gazed at my beloved wife again, and even though I was no longer scared, I realised I mustn't look at her any more. I had to go on, had to keep strong for Ryan and Reece and Damon, had to go home and be strong for the five little ones as well, had to tell them all the worst thing a child could ever hear. And, to be strong enough to do that, I knew I mustn't look at Angie's body any longer. I needed the image in my head to be the right one: the one of the happy smiling woman I loved. Not looking like this. Without her smile she didn't look like Angie any more.

'Take me home,' I said to Malc. 'I need to be with the kids now.'

Eileen drives us home and Malc gets out of the car with me.

'I'll stay with you,' he tells me. 'I'll make a cup of tea, lad.'

I go into the living room and sit down in the armchair by the front window and stare sightlessly out while he does so.

The tea made, he comes and joins me, taking a seat in the other armchair, but still we sit in silence as there's nothing to say. Every time I so much as edge towards thinking about life without her, I break down. It's as if my body was no longer under my control.

Malc looks on, lets me cry. 'I don't know what to say to you,' he tells me. Which makes something jolt in me.

'I have to tell Herbert,' I say, remembering. 'I have to go down and tell him. He didn't even know she was in hospital.'

'I'll come with you,' Malc says, rising from his chair along with me.

I shake my head.

'No,' I say. 'I need to do this myself.'

But, as I walk down the road to his bungalow, I see his bedroom curtains are still drawn, and, when I try the door, it's double-locked. I'll have to come back, I decide, and turn around to head back home, but, as I do so, one of my friends, Dean, who lives on our street, comes down his front path and beckons me across the road. News travels fast; clearly. Dean's married to a friend of my nephew Adrian's wife and I know he texted her while still at the hospital. That's obviously how Dean knows.

'Ian, mate,' he says. 'I'm so sorry about Angie. Come on, come on in for a bit. Andrea wants to talk to you.'

Dean's wife has just finished a course of chemotherapy for breast cancer herself, so I know Angie's death will be particularly hard for her. She puts her arms around me and hugs me tightly. 'I just can't believe it,' she says. 'I only saw her in the garden yesterday. She looked fine then.'

I tell her I'm as shocked as she is. But I'm still not all there. My mind's still on Herbert and the job I have to do. But when I leave their house the curtains on the bungalow are still drawn so I have no choice but to go back to Malc. 'You know,' I say, 'I used to think Angie's dad was lucky, living so long and being so fit, but there's nothing lucky about living to ninety-one only to have your wife and youngest daughter die within twenty-one days of each other, is there?'

I'm dreading telling him, but, till I do, I don't seem to be able to do anything else, so I try again, at eight – it's turned out to be a beautiful sunny morning – and I can see him smiling at me from the front window. I smile back automatically, but, as soon as I'm inside and he's sitting down in his favourite armchair, I kneel in front of him, take his hand, and burst into tears.

'It's Angie,' I say brokenly. 'She's died.'

He says nothing for a long time. Just stares into the depths of the roaring coal fire he's already made, then he turns and looks at his hand, which I still have pressed to my cheek. 'Oh, our Angie,' he says quietly, his eyes glistening with unshed tears. 'Oh, Angie. She was such a jolly lass.'

Which makes me cry even more. Why Angie? Why her? Why take someone who had so much love for life?

'I know how hard this is, lad,' Herbert's saying, 'because I know how much you two loved each other. But if there's anything you need, anything, you just ask me, okay?' And I know he means it. I've been so lucky – doubly blessed in having Angie. I didn't just get the girl of my dreams, I got another set of loving parents as well. It's no surprise my wife's always been such an incredible woman. I just have to look where she came from to know why.

Herbert takes me to the door and as I leave he says it again. Anything. Anything at all that he can do for me. And, even though there's nothing I need except the one thing I can't have, I've never been more grateful for his love.

Malc goes home once I'm back, to see how Eileen is. In the middle of everything she's been feeling really sick and he needs to get home and check she's okay. He's reluctant to leave me but I promise him I'll be okay. The kids are sleeping over at Damon and Natalie's, and Reece is round at Ryan's, so the house is now empty. And, for the moment at least, it's the way I need it to be. If I'm going to fall apart, and I know I am, it's better that I'm alone.

And I do fall apart, utterly. How the hell am I going to tell the kids? It's such a terrifying thing to contemplate that I decide then and there that there is no way in the world that I can tell them today. I don't have the strength. I'm not sure I have the strength to even get through today, let alone the rest of my life – *our* lives. Where do you begin? Everywhere I look, there she is. In every photo, smiling out at me, looking so happy. And the echo of her presence fills every corner of our house. I wander the rooms, racked with tears, suffocated by the memory of her presence, and when I go into our bedroom, see the clothes I had to change her out of, see the indentation in the pillow where she'd lain only yesterday, I feel so much pain it's as if my heart had been ripped out.

Reece and Sophie arrive home around nine and being forced to pull myself together is hard but necessary. I am in such a state that it feels as if I am hanging by a thread and, though we talk little, their presence is like a safety rope, hauling me back.

I find enough presence of mind, at least, to call Damon and let him know what I've decided. That I'll hold off telling the little ones that Angie's gone till tomorrow, because I cannot – I *must* not – fall apart when I do. Damon agrees, and says they'll just tell them Angie's still in hospital and that they don't have to go to school today and leave it at that.

But, when he and Nat arrive home at noon with the children, I find it almost impossible to bear. Having made the decision not to tell them, I can hardly bear to look at them. Every time I catch a glimpse of their smiling, happy faces it reminds me of the terrible enormity of their loss, and provokes another rush of hot, shuddering sobs. I have to get out, in the end, because I feel like I can't breathe, and if I fall apart in front of them I know they will be terrified.

I put Angie's soiled clothes in the washing machine and run it, then, with Sophie and Natalie taking charge – they are such wonderful girls, both of them – I go outside and climb into the car. I start driving, even though I don't know where to drive to. But something leads me to the cemetery where we laid Winnie to rest just a couple of weeks back. I don't know why, but being close to Winnie feels like the right thing to do. Thank God she didn't have to bear Angie's death at least. The grave is still covered in floral tributes, including mine and Angie's. The card's still there too – it reads, TO A WONDERFUL LOVING MUM. GONE FROM OUR HOME BUT NOT OUR HEARTS. There's no headstone yet, of course: it's only been a couple of weeks since we got a book of headstone styles for Herbert to choose from, and since Angie asked me to bring her up here, too, so she could see if there was anything she particularly liked.

And she had: she'd seen one that she thought would be perfect. It looked like the Gates of Heaven, with black and gold lettering. Herbert hadn't agreed, though, and, in the end, it was his decision. He'd opted for a heart one instead.

I look at the flowers. Look at the grass beside the freshly covered grave. The Gates of Heaven will sit well here. Because Angie will have them. And the knowledge that she's going to is a comfort. But it's the tiniest scrap of comfort in a violent storm of pain. I kneel down beside Winnie's grave and cry and cry and cry. I can't believe the plot I bought for myself just twenty-one days ago is going to be opened up so soon.

When I leave the cemetery, I go down to see the funeral director. He's surprised, although not *that* surprised, to see me again so soon, because he naturally thinks I'm here for a different reason.

'Is it about Winnie's funeral?' he asks me, confused, as he shows me in. I don't blame him. What other reason *would* he think I'd have to be there?

When I explain, he suggests I leave arranging everything for a couple of days yet, but I can't bear to. I need to do this now and I need to do it properly. I order the very best of everything, everything I know Angie wanted from her own mother's funeral, including the beautiful carved Last Supper coffin – which was so lovely it moved Angie to tears – and, fittingly, the Gates of Heaven headstone for her grave.

At least she's with her mum now.

I don't sleep a wink that first night. I don't even try to. I can't even bear to go into our bedroom, because I know I'll just keep seeing the dent in the pillow where Angie's head should be. Instead, once Damon and Nat have gone home with Warren, and Reece and Sophie have gone to bed, I huddle on the sofa, with the television on, watching the pictures flicker past me but not seeing any of them. Instead my eyes keep being drawn to the photos we have everywhere, particularly the canvas of the Valentine's Day photograph the photo-processing shop did for us, which now has such painful significance.

I keep being drawn back to that step in the park, too – *our* step – and at one point even contemplate walking there. How did we get from there to this in such a scarily short time? It feels so much as if all that happened just yesterday. Where's my life gone? Where has Angie's? What happens now?

Unsurprisingly, when dawn finally comes to release me, I go through the morning rituals on feet that feel like lead. I can see the weight of grief pressing down on Reece, too. He's being so brave, holding himself together, and being so strong for the little ones. I'm so proud of him and the thought of how proud Angie would be of him too gives me a shot in the arm I so badly need.

Sophie's being an angel, too – she and Natalie always have been. And she's taking care of both of us by taking charge of the children, bless her – getting them up and dressed, organising breakfast and so on, because I'm useless and have to keep out of their way. Though I try to keep it together, I am on the edge of tears, constantly struggling to stop myself breaking down.

The younger children, oblivious, are excitable and playful – they love having Sophie staying, and to them the day's a special one. They can't believe their luck: they're going to get the rest of the week off school, and can spend it playing Xbox and watching telly – which, though it can't be helped, makes the task seem even more insurmountable. Every time I look in on them, all together in the living room, I get so choked up seeing them so happy and carefree that I know I won't be able to speak. The thought that they don't know they no longer have a mummy overwhelms me to the point of almost paralysing me. Never have I so badly wanted to run away from something – as if I were a little child myself.

But I have to be strong. I can already hear Angie chastising me. Telling me to keep myself together while I tell them. Do it for *me*, Mill. Be their rock. Tell them without shedding a single tear. Because, if *you* fall apart, then so will their world. And she's right. I *am* their world now. What else do they have to cling to, if not me?

Returning to the kitchen for a third time, I stand and stare out of the window, and I'm still trying to stem my tears when I become aware that someone's come into the kitchen. I turn around to see Connor, his expression anxious. He's eleven now. He understands things. He knows something terrible has happened. He just doesn't know what yet.

'Come here,' I say, beckoning to him. 'There's something I need to tell you.'

As soon as he's level with me, I drop to my knees in front of him, so we're eye to eye, and place my hands on his shoulders. 'Connor, love,' I tell him. 'I'm so sorry – your mum died last night.'

I watch his eyes fill with tears, his worst imaginings all come true now. 'I know, Dad,' he says. 'I heard you and Reece talking about it last night.'

Reece comes in just as I'm crushing Connor against me, and I realise I have to finish this job right now. Reece stays and comforts Connor while I go into the living room to tell the other children. Dodging their toys, I go and sit down on the sofa, behind where they're all clustered on the floor in front of the television, and will myself to dam the ever-threatening tears.

'Hey, kids,' I say. They turn around almost as one. 'Come and sit beside me,' I say to them. 'I want to tell you something.'

Being kids – and happy kids, because they're their mum's kids, because she lives in them – they scramble up excitedly, as if I were going to tell them something fun. Jake and Jade snuggle up on one side of me and Corey and Ella take a knee each, and it breaks my heart to see all their faces angled towards me so expectantly, and to know the agony of what lies ahead.

I turn to Jake and Jade. 'You know your mum's been very ill, don't you?' They nod in unison.

'Yes,' Jade says. 'When's she coming home, Dad?'

Try as I might to stop them, the tears are rolling freely down my cheeks now. 'She's not coming home, love,' I manage to say. 'She's died. She's up in Heaven now.'

Within the blink of an eye, Jake and Jade are crying with

me, and almost immediately Corey starts wailing too. It's only Ella – tiny Ella – who's dry-eyed. She just sits on my knee, smiling beatifically up at me, smiling Angie's smile, her mother's precious gift.

She looks awed, in fact. 'So is Mummy an angel now?' she asks me.

I nod, clasping the children to me as tightly as I can, for strength. 'Yes,' I say, 'she is, and she'll be looking down from Heaven and watching you. Watching *all* of you,' I tell them, 'and she doesn't want to see you sad. If *you're* sad, then Mummy's sad, but, if she sees you smiling, *she'll* be smiling. So we have to do the best we can, so that Mummy can see us smiling. Okay? Let's try to make your mum happy.'

Chapter 19

I have to pick up Angie's death certificate at the hospital the following day, and I'm absolutely dreading going back there. But, at the same time, I'm being pulled there by my need to find out why she died so suddenly. It's been playing on my mind endlessly – how can she have been so well that morning and dead before the following night was out? The more I think about it, the more I have this terrible sense of things not being right somehow. How could she be so full of life one minute and dead the next? *How?*

It's still a struggle, though, as I walk down the corridor to the registrar's office. It's the same corridor I ran along after Jonathan came out to find me, and retracing my steps makes the hairs prickle at the back of my neck. It makes me remember things I can't bear to remember, and see things I don't want to see.

I don't have to wait long till the registrar comes out. He takes me into his office, tells me to sit down and then offers me his condolences. He then pulls a folder out of a drawer in his desk and removes a piece of paper from it.

'Here we are,' he says, sliding the document across the desk to me. 'You just need to sign this form for me, Mr Millthorpe, then take it down to the Town Hall in order to register your wife's death.' He passes me a pen. 'Then they'll give you the death certificate.'

I take the form from him. 'Thank you,' I say. 'But can you tell me *how* she died?'

He looks confused. Then slides the form back, then says, 'Cancer. Your wife died from cancer, Mr Millthorpe.'

I feel overtaken by a sudden surge of anger, hearing this. 'You can't tell me it was the cancer that killed her,' I argue. 'She was fine the day I brought her into the hospital – she was cleaning the house the morning she died. She was even laughing and joking in the car when I brought her here. So don't try telling me the cancer killed her, because it didn't!'

The registrar stares at me, obviously shocked by what I've said to him – and at my tone, as well – and I feel guilty that I've raised my voice. Then he frowns. 'Well, if that's the case,' he says, 'I think you'd better speak to the coroner. Tell him what you've just told me.'

Feeling calmer now, I tell him I'm happy to do that, so he dials a number and gets through to someone – I presume the coroner – and tells him I don't agree with what's been put down as the cause of Angie's death. Then he hands me the phone. I take it.

It *is* the coroner. 'Why is it that you think your wife didn't die from her cancer?' he wants to know. So I tell him what I told the registrar, just as I've been told to. 'Well, in that case,' he says, 'we'll need to carry out a postmortem in order that we can definitely ascertain the cause of death. Are you happy for us to do that?'

Despite the chain of events I seem to have put in motion, I feel repulsed by the idea of a stranger touching Angie's body. She's been through so much – how can I allow them to put her through more? 'No,' I say. 'You can't do that. I'm not letting anyone touch her.'

'Mr Millthorpe,' the coroner says patiently. 'If you allow us to do a postmortem, we'll be able to tell you what killed your wife. If you don't, however – if you leave this till after the funeral's taken place – we won't be able to do that, and you'll have to live with not knowing. So,' he finishes, 'think about it carefully. How about I give you ten minutes to think about it and then call you back? Would that be an idea?'

I tell him yes, but as I hand the phone back to the registrar I feel the same sense of revulsion at the idea of strangers touching Angie's body. Yes, I want to know what happened, but what right do I have to let them do that to her? Would that be what *she'd* want?

I explain to the registrar what the coroner said to me, and, as we wait for the call, I repeat what I said to him. 'I can't let them do that to her,' I tell him, shaking my head. 'And that's that.'

The registrar is very sympathetic and I feel sorry that I was angry with him. But he also thinks I'm wrong to refuse the postmortem. 'Mr Millthorpe,' he says gently, 'you know, if I were you, I'd let them carry it out. If you don't, it'll be playing on your mind for the rest of your life.'

I know he's right. I know it would eat me up, not know-ing. Angie's been dead only days and it's already eating me up. I can't let it lie. My brain just won't let me. So when the coroner calls back, exactly ten minutes later, I tell him they can do the postmortem.

'You've made the right decision,' he says. But have I?

The registrar then gives me a white plastic bag, fastened with a tie-wrap, which he tells me contains Angie's clothes. And, as I walk back down the corridor, all I can think about is how close to me my dear wife is at this moment, lying in the hospital morgue. I can't think beyond that. Right or wrong, it just feels horrible.

The next few days are a blur of grief, days that seem to melt into one another, as the waves of distress keep overtaking me. I've never been more grateful for having such a big and loving family than I am now. Though I feel I'm stumbling through each hour, trying not to break down in front of the little ones, there's a constant reassuring presence of family in the house – people who loved Angie and know just what a huge hole she's left in our lives, and who cook and shop and tidy and entertain the children, at what feels like all hours of the day and night.

I don't think it's really sunk in yet for the little ones. Where Reece's and Connor's grief is etched so clearly in their faces, the younger ones seem in a state of suspended animation. Constantly occupied, as they are, by a loving procession of relatives, for them it seems to feel more like an unexpected holiday. And, though I know this state is temporary, and that when it does hit them, they will be devastated, I'm grateful for this temporary respite.

My sister Karen comes most days, with her daughter, my niece Julie. Julie's a mum herself now, with two teenagers, Jodi and Jake, and the girls love it when she comes because she gives them both makeovers. And though it's painful to watch, as Julie carefully applies nail polish to Jade's fingers, I'm so glad they have all these wonderful women in their lives.

Ella's fascinated by the nail polish. 'I want some,' she says to Julie. 'I want some Ella polish too!'

Julie smiles at her. 'That's a good name,' she says to Ella. 'Much better than nail polish, isn't it?'

And, as Ella holds her tiny fingers out to await her turn to have some 'Ella polish', I just hope Angie's watching. Hope she knows her little girls will be okay.

On the Monday I decide to take the children back to school. They need to be back with their friends, and back in some sort of routine, to start the inch-by-inch process of adapting to their new future, coming to terms with losing their mum and rebuilding their lives. Reece, too, returns to routine, having been given the week off work, and at least the days will have some structure once again.

As I help the little ones wash and dress – aided by Sophie, who's staying for the fortnight – I feel my stomach churning at the thought of arriving at the school gates, because I know everyone's going to want to talk to me about Angie, and I'm not sure I'm strong enough to cope with it without cracking up.

I'm also aware that I'm already failing.

'Can't you do a plait, Daddy?' Jade says, as we stand in front of the lounge mirror and I start gathering her hair into a ponytail.

'I'm sorry, love,' I say. 'I don't have enough time to do a plait today.'

As soon as I say it, I realise it's something Angie would never have said to her. And I can see in her eyes she knows that too. But the truth is, I can't do it. Not properly. I'm not good enough yet. Angie wasn't supposed to *die* yet. I'm still all fingers and thumbs.

'You should teach me,' says Jade. 'Then I can do it myself. And after that,' she says, 'you can teach me to French-plait as well. And then I can do Ella's hair, and then you'll have more time to do everything, won't you?'

I feel like my heart's ripping in two. 'This afternoon,' I tell her. 'I promise.'

Sure enough, as soon as we arrive at school, we're ambushed by people, mostly women, wanting to tell us how sorry they are to hear that Angie has gone. Jake and Jade look ashen, like two haunted wraiths amid all the boisterousness of the play-ground, Jade clutching my hand as if she dare not let me go. I'm overwhelmed by how many people come to pay their respects, but, even so, I'm glad to escape and take the twins to their classrooms, and then get to the relative sanctuary of the nursery unit.

It's while I'm in there, hanging up Corey's coat, that Teresa, the nursery nurse, comes over. I don't mind facing her: as well as being one of Corey's teachers, she's also a good friend.

'Ian,' she says, 'you know we've had so many people coming into reception this past week, wanting to know when Angie's funeral's going to be. So I was wondering, would it be okay with you if we sent a letter home with the children today or tomorrow, letting them know what the funeral arrangements are?'

I'm so touched. I haven't really thought beyond friends and family, but then I realise Angie had so *many* friends – as she would, because everyone loved her. I tell Teresa where it'll be, and that I'll call and let them know when I have the date, and feel choked up to think they're going to do that, all the way home.

And it's almost as if Angie's been watching over me while this is happening, and knows I'm only hanging on by a thread. Because, as soon as I get in, the house phone rings. It's the funeral director, calling to tell me she's there with them at last, and that I can come and see her any time I like.

'And is this Thursday at eleven thirty going to be okay with you for the funeral?' he asks me.

I tell him yes. Though all I can think of right now is that I can now go and see Angie. It's been five days now, and I miss her so much. And, now I know she's at rest, seeing her holds no fears.

And I'm right. Angie looks so beautiful and peaceful, lying in her polished dark-oak coffin, her hair just as lustrous and shiny as the sheen on the wood. Her hand is cold when I pick it up and lift it to my cheek, but it's still *her* hand, its contours as familiar as my own. I sit for an hour with her, holding her hand and stroking her hair, and, though I'm crying, I'm so glad to have this time alone with her.

The following day I get a visit from my friend Dave and his wife, Chris. I've known him since we were boys – in fact, we all went to school together – and he and I were born on the same day. He's brought a sympathy card and asks what day the funeral is going to be, and when I tell him Thursday he has a shocked look on his face.

'Thursday?' he says. 'Didn't you realise Thursday is your birthday?'

I can't believe what I've done, that the date didn't register. But it's too late to do anything about it. I've already phoned the school and the letters have gone out to the parents now, so it seems I'll just have to bury Angie on my birthday. But a part of me doesn't care anyway. I'm going to love her till my dying day, after all, so why wouldn't I want to remember her on my birthday?

In the meantime, however, I have two precious days left with her. The older boys don't want to visit, because they want to remember their mum as she was in life, and I understand that: seeing a person you love in death is very harrowing. But for me it's like a lifeline, seeing my beautiful wife finally at peace and out of pain.

And, when the time comes for me to leave her on the Wednesday afternoon, it hits me hard that our time together – on earth, at least – is almost up. I've brought photographs of all the children and tuck them in close beside her. I've also decided to bury her wearing her jewellery. She loved her rings, so it seems only right that she should take them with her, as well as the favourite gold chain she liked to wear round her neck. I've brought another ring for her to take with her as well: when Winnie died, Herbert gave Angie one of her rings – a wishbone ring that belonged to her grandmother. Angie's not yet worn it because it was too large and kept slipping off her finger. I slip it on there now, where it belongs.

And then I find I can't leave. I'm rooted to the spot. I keep trying to, but, every time I kiss her goodbye and turn to go, it hits me that this will be the last time I'll ever see her face, and though I eventually make it to the door – three separate times, maybe four – I look back at her and can't seem to turn away again. I have to keep going back to give her one last kiss.

It feels exactly as it did when we were courting and saying goodnight. One last kiss. One last goodbye. One last cuddle. Except this time it's not just till tomorrow: it's forever.

I lean in to kiss her again. 'I'll always love you, Angie,' I whisper. And this time, when I get to the door of the chapel, I hurry out, without looking back.

Chapter 20

As soon as I see the first hearse drive up the road, I know it's an image that will haunt me for the rest of my life. The sleek car is the first of two that are arriving; another has been brought just to hold all the floral tributes that have been sent. Following behind them are three shiny limousines for the family, their black bodywork reflecting the leaden skies above. But it's the first car that transfixes me as I stare out of the window. Numb with grief, feeling sick, I can't take my eyes from it, because, as I watch its slow and steady progress towards our home, I realise that this flower-filled car carries my childhood sweetheart, Angie, my most treasured possession.

The vicar had been to see me on the Tuesday. He obviously wanted to talk to me about Angie, so that he could speak about her as part of the service. I made him a cup of tea and took him into the living room to talk, and straightaway I could see what a wise man he was, because almost the first thing he said to me was something that I'd never even thought of.

'You know, Ian,' he said, 'maybe the fact that Angie was

destined to die at such a young age is the reason the two of you found each other as young as you did.'

I hadn't thought of it like that before. Instead of seeing things in terms of just how much time we'd had together, I could think only in terms of how much time we now *wouldn't* have. But it *has* been a long time – compared with many couples, we've been lucky. I've had Angie to love for a full thirty-five years.

The vicar also wanted to know how we met, so I told him about Angie's mate asking if I'd go on a date with her, and how, even though it was a filthy afternoon – dark and cold and raining stair rods – for me it was as if the sun had come out. I'd been so happy, I didn't care that I got soaked. I'd sung to myself all the way home.

'How about hymns?' he wanted to know next. 'Favourite songs she had and so on.' And I told him I'd like them to play 'Rule the World' by Take That. Angie loved all the boy bands, and particularly that track, after hearing it played at Stephen Gately's funeral.

'And "You Raise Me Up" by Westlife,' I told him. 'For when we leave the church.'

I knew that would be perfect, and it was another one I'd already decided on, not just because we both loved it but also because it summed up everything about what Angie meant to me. She always made me feel more than I could ever be.

Just as he was leaving, the vicar pointed to the big canvas picture in the living room, the one they'd done for us when they damaged the film from our anniversary trip.

'When did you have that done?' he asked.

'We didn't,' I told him. 'It's just a blow-up of a snap we had from Valentine's Day 2005 that Angie always had on her bedside table.'

I explained about what had happened to all the pictures from Llandudno. 'That's such a shame,' the vicar said. 'But this is lovely. Perhaps we could put it beside Angie's coffin. What do you think?'

I told him I thought it would be lovely if we could do that. Inasmuch as I could think about it all. Mostly, I couldn't bear to.

Angie's funeral is to take place in St Luke's Church in Grimethorpe, the church where she was christened in 1962, and where we were married in 1985 – though we should have been wed a year earlier. We were both working now, and had been saving hard, ready for our wedding, as well as putting things away for our bottom drawer. There being no jobs around in nursery nursing, Angie had a job as a cleaner at Barnsley Hospital, and I was now a face worker at the colliery, driving the shearer, the machine that runs along the coal face. So life was good, the time was right, and we had the date booked and everything, but then the miners' strike happened and everything had to be put on hold.

We'd been devastated to have to wait to get married. Who wouldn't be? We'd been together ten years and couldn't wait to make a home together, Angie particularly. She couldn't wait to be a bride and start a family. It was all she'd ever wanted. But there was no question of going ahead with it till the strike was over. As was the case for every mining community back in that dark, dark year, the people in Grimethorpe really struggled to get by, and every penny was required just to exist on the basics; there was nothing spare for putting on fancy things like weddings.

It was a grim time for the whole community, but we coped. There was nothing else to do, and no money coming in, either, so, when we weren't manning the picket lines (an angry, volatile and dispiriting business), we made what we could by picking coal off the colliery's muck tip, and selling it by the sack to those who most needed it – mostly elderly people who couldn't get coal because of the strike, and who were just so grateful to have any at all. It was punishing work, made worse by such a red-hot summer, but at least it got us through the endless months without pay.

Not that we came out of it with anything positive. If anything, the future looked bleaker. It felt as if the whole community had endured twelve months of struggle for nothing. We were solid in Grimethorpe, though, because mining was our and our children's future, and we didn't know anything else. So, when we were instructed to return to work, having achieved nothing but heartache, we felt that the union – the union that had put us through so much – had caved in and really let us down.

But, whatever I didn't have, I had the one thing that mattered more than anything: I had my Angie, and at last we could be wed.

The Valentine's Day picture is one of the first things I see as I enter St Luke's, supported by my three oldest boys. But it's not the very first. As we walk up the aisle behind the pall-bearers carrying Angie's coffin what transfixes me most is the sheer number of people crammed in there. I'm shocked to see that not only is every seat filled, but every inch of standing room is also taken. I can't believe how many people – many of whom I don't even recognise – have come to join us in paying their respects. I'm so touched that they've bothered to do this – to say goodbye to this fellow mum they'd see on the school run every morning, pushing a child in a pram, with a long line of children following behind her, and always – as one woman says to me – *always* smiling.

I have decided against bringing the younger children to the funeral. They're all so young, and it will be much too distressing for them to be here. So my neighbour is looking after them, and, as we take our places, I know it was the right decision: I can barely keep my legs from buckling under me, and I know Angie would hate them to see me like this.

The service itself is to be a traditional one. Though I can't get a note out, the congregation sing 'Jerusalem', and the sound of their voices completely fills the space. Out of all those voices, however, I pick out just one: the powerful yet beautiful tones of my Uncle Bill, who spent many years singing in a male-voice choir.

Uncle Bill's married to Rose, my mum's younger sister, and they, too, have had life deal them a cruel blow. They had only the one son, our Anthony, but they lost him in 1975, just before he was due to get wed. He worked at Shafton Workshops, repairing the machinery we used down the mines, and had changed his shift one day so he could visit the solicitor and sort out something to do with the house he and his fiancée were buying. He then went into work for the afternoon shift instead, and was crushed between two pieces of machinery.

Listening to Bill – who adored Angie – and remembering my cousin Anthony does help to pull me together. My heart is broken, but I had twenty-five years married to Angie. Anthony had none, and Bill and Rose lost their only child.

But the vicar seems to know how Angie would have wanted him to play it, because, the hymn done and us sitting again, he shocks everyone by bursting into song. He clears his throat and starts to belt out the opening bars of 'Singin' in the Rain'.

'I bet you're all wondering,' he says, to an open-mouthed congregation, 'why I'm singing such a happy song at a funeral.' He then recounts how it had been raining on the day I found out that Angie wanted to go out with me, and how that had been exactly the way I'd felt – '. . . and has continued to feel, though their long and happy marriage,' I hear him saying. I'm listening, but I'm numb. I can't think straight.

The journey from the church to the cemetery takes only a few minutes, and, sitting in the back of the funeral car with the boys and Nat and Sophie, I'm dreading what now lies ahead. I think we all are. Few words are exchanged. Mostly, we just stare, locked in our own thoughts, out of the windows, watching an indifferent world spool before our eyes. Though not always indifferent: I'm touched to see a gang of hoodies, when they see us, stop what they're doing, lower their hoods and bow their heads with respect. We also pass the house Angie grew up in, and, just before it, the very same corner the vicar was referring to: the place where her mate asked me if I'd go on a date with her. The pain of remembering that day is palpable.

We hold the wake in the Grimethorpe Working Men's Club, as we did Winnie's, and, once again, I'm overwhelmed by the sheer number of people. There must be in excess of two hundred crammed in there, and I try my best to speak to those I can. It's really hard though, and I go through the motions in a kind of fog. All I really want to do is run away.

I pick the little ones up as soon as we're home, at around two. That's it, I think. We've got through it. We're done. I feel relieved that it's over, but at the same time anxious: what now? The thought that I now have to get on with the rest of my life is so scary I want to run away and hide from it; I keep feeling panicky to know how much my children now depend on me, how they will look to me for everything now their mum's no longer here.

All the close members of the family have come home with me. As well as all the boys and their girlfriends there are Malc and Eileen, Karen and her brother Arthur, as well as Glenn, who I know will be my rock over the coming weeks, and has promised me he'll help me through the early days.

'You just say what you need doing,' he reassures me. 'And I'll be there. And, if you need to go out, just you phone me and I'll be right up to look after them.' It's such a comfort to know he's there because the children all adore him, and I know his reassuring presence will make everything that bit better for them.

I'm also grateful to have him in my life. One thing that I'm clear on is that it's just me and the kids now. The thought of another woman coming into their lives and spending time with them that should have been Angie's is an idea I can't imagine ever being able to stomach.

But, much as I'm grateful to have my brothers and sisters around me, the day's taken its toll and I'm struggling. Everywhere I look I'm reminded that she's gone, and, now the funeral is over, I feel worse than ever. I go upstairs into our bedroom, thinking I'll find some solace there, but seeing her side of the bed feels like a physical pain. How will I ever be able to sleep in this room again? And, having no sense of smell, I can't even gather up her clothes and drink her scent in. I don't even have that much to hang onto. All I have left of her is the single lock of hair that I had Angie's sister-in-law Diane cut for me when she went to say goodbye yesterday evening. I sit on the bed and open the little silver box that Diane put it in. And, as I touch it with my finger, I'm grateful that at least Angie didn't lose her hair again. It's only a crumb of comfort, but at least it's something.

I close the box again, feeling the pain welling in me. So, realising that I'm going to struggle now not to fall apart in front of the children, I go back downstairs and ask Reece and Damon if they'll take charge for a while so I can drive back to the cemetery to spend some time alone at Angie's grave.

When I get there I'm shocked anew at just how many

flowers there are around it. It's a dazzlingly bright display compared with the dull autumn tones of the cemetery – almost like an expression of her own beauty. As well as my own wreath, which says WIFE, with a posy of red roses, there's a beautiful one from Ryan – an open book, with a picture of Angie in the middle – the Gates of Heaven, the big white one that spells out AUNTIE ANGIE in tiny flowers, and the children's huge letters, spelling MUMMY.

I don't feel able to read the words on any of the cards, my own included, so I purposely don't try to. I simply stand there and look. But it's not long before I realise I can't stay here anyway. I know I'll be coming back here – to my dying day, all the while my legs can still carry me – but right now Angie's presence here, deep under the ground, is too harrowing. I know I need to be somewhere else.

It doesn't take me long to realise where that somewhere is. I drive straight to the park and climb out of the car, pulling my jacket tighter around me. It's not dark yet, but the day's been a gloomy one, and I see almost no one as I go in. I pass an elderly couple walking a dog as I head up to the pavilion and, painfully, a couple of teenagers, boy and girl, hand in hand. They're in school uniform. Like an echo of our own past. I can't look at them.

When I get to the pavilion, which is closed up for the winter now, I sit down on our step, the setting for our very first date. I put a hand out and touch it, feel the cold of the stone seeping into me, remember how Angie would comment on it every single time we passed it. 'That's our step that is, Mill,' she'd say. Then she'd smile.

And it's while I'm sitting there – on our step – that, for the first time today, I remember that it's my forty-ninth birthday. I'm forty-nine and I'm alone. I am a widower. The word rolls around my head, jangly and alien. A *widower*. How can I ever go on without her?

It's a horrible dark time, and my head is suddenly full of the sorts of thoughts that frighten me – thoughts I know I have to fight to push away. I've lost my soulmate, and I know there is a simple solution to my terrible pain: if I were to die too, it would be gone and we would be reunited. It's the simplicity of it that makes it so compelling. The future is just too impossible a thing to contemplate; in comparison, death seems so much easier. Easier for everyone. After all, what use am I going to be to my children when I can barely get through the day?

But I do chase the thoughts away, because other voices in my head are louder. The voice of sanity, temporarily displaced by a kind of madness; and Angie's voice too, which was always going to be the strongest, the one that reminds me that I made her a promise to do my best to bring the kids up, to take her place. Which reminds me of something else: what use is Heaven with Angie if I get there before I'm supposed to, and she turns away from me because I've already failed her? My children have already lost their mother. They need their father now more than ever. Our children. *Angie's* children. I can't let her down now, not after all the hard work she's put into making sure I can look after them without her. Life *has* to go on, however painful it's going to be. And I have to trust that the pain will get easier.

The sky's darkening as I stand up and take one last lingering look at the park around me, at the view we've gazed out on together for thirty-five long years, the place where so many of my most cherished memories have been made, the place where the spirit of my dead wife is always going to be. Then I walk back to the car and drive home to my children, who are now my life and my most important responsibility.

Chapter 21

I keep the children off school again the day after the funeral, so that we can all go and say goodbye to their mum while it's still light. Once again we pass the home where she lived when we were courting, and I'm comforted to know she's so close.

Corey and Ella are excited to see so many flowers for their mummy, and by the fact that, when people pass the grave they stop to look, but we don't stay long because, for the older three, it's just so upsetting. As it would be: there is a whole world of difference between visiting the grave of an elderly grandma and visiting that of your mum – who was, for the younger children, their whole world and who is now buried underneath the ground.

Though I wouldn't wish what has happened to my children on my worst enemy, there is a part of me that's grateful that the littlest ones, at least, have so little sense of the enormity of what they've lost. And it's clear they don't. Though Corey, almost five now, is obviously aware of his brothers' and older sister's distress, little Ella is oblivious. While we huddle together against the cold, clinging to one another, I can sense her confusion about everyone's sadness.

It also really brings it home to me how unfair this all seems. Much as I know there is no plan to who lives and who dies, being with my children, visiting Angie's grave, feels all wrong. It should be Angie standing here with them, not I. It's the wrong way round. If one of us had to die, then it should have been I. It should be she – their selfless, adoring and brilliant mother – who guides them through the dark times and watches them grow and blossom, who gets the reward for all those years of care and love. In the short term it should be she watching them open their presents come Christmas. It's just wrong on every level. So undeserved.

We don't linger. There will be other times, when everyone's less fragile, and, when I ask the children if they want to go home now, I can see the relief on the faces of the older three.

Ella is happy to go now in any case. She's impatient to move on to something else, as toddlers always are. 'See ya later, Mummy!' she chirrups as I gather her up to leave. Her little hand waves from side to side, just as Angie taught her. 'Byee!' she goes. 'Bye, Mummy. See ya soon!'

I'm emotionally drained now, from trying to keep strong, and every day brings its own triggers, moments when the sight of something, sound of something or just an unbidden memory creeps up and knocks me for six.

I can't help but know that Angie would just be so much better than me at this; that, were we to swap places, she'd find reserves of strength I don't have. I keep thinking back to the words of that Westlife song that meant so much to us.

Without her I seem to be sinking and sinking – all my own strength just seems to have ebbed away.

On the Monday after the funeral, I get a poignant reminder of the truth in that. It's mid-afternoon, and Ella's gone to Nat's. To give me a break, she's taken her there for the day, to play with Warren.

Not that I've achieved much as yet: I've taken the dogs to the woods for a walk, and I've looked in on Herbert, but I'm just standing at the kitchen window, looking out on nothing, when I hear the squeak of the kitchen door opening.

It's Reece and Sophie. They're both home, because Reece has got the week off work. His boss has been kind to him and Damon, for which I'm grateful. Reece is holding something, something wrapped that looks like a present – a present he's now holding out to me.

And it is. 'Dad, here's your birthday present,' he says.

I'm so moved, but at the same time my heart sinks. I asked the children not to get me cards or presents for my birthday. It was the last thing I wanted, both for me and for them. How could anyone celebrate a birthday right now?

'Oh, Reece,' I say, 'I told you not to . . .'

But he's shaking his head. 'It's your present from Mum,' he explains. 'She gave me the money to get it for you.' He gives it to me. 'Just last month. Just the weekend before she died.'

Reece is struggling to get the words out, but is just about holding himself together. Sophie, I notice, holds his hand for support. I'm so glad he has her. Glad my older boys all have girls to take care of them.

I open the parcel and inside I find a box containing a

satnav. 'She wanted to give it to you for your birthday, Dad,' Reece adds. 'Only . . .' He falters, then stops. Then, perhaps realising I'm going to fall apart at any moment, he and Sophie turn around and leave the kitchen.

I don't do as well at holding up as my brave son. I am moved to tears, the grief completely hijacking me. And, with Reece and Sophie gone, I break down again completely, and it's a real effort of will to get myself together again in time to drive up to school to collect the others. The same question keeps coming back to me. Why did she die like that? Why so suddenly? Why okay one minute and the next in the morgue?

Receiving the satnav just seems to crystallise my thinking. I'm not going to find peace till I find out what happened. This was supposed to be for our trip to Llandudno, this satnav. Angie had bought it to help guide us back to the holiday we would never now take. And I just can't get my head around why she died so unexpectedly. It makes no more sense to me than it did at the time – less now, if anything. I just can't believe the cancer could have killed her so suddenly.

I knew she was dying – of course I did – but why in this way? Why so unexpectedly? I am desperate for answers, and I need to try to find some, and I've not yet heard anything about the result of the postmortem. I decide to call the hospital and get put through to Lynne Handley of PALS, and she tells me she'll get an appointment made for me with Angie's oncologist.

'And I'll come with you,' she says, when she calls back,

having made one for the following Thursday. And I'm touched, because Lynne finishes work at 4.30, and the appointment's not till the consultant finishes her clinic at 6 p.m.

But it's not a productive encounter. 'What the hell went wrong?' I want to know as soon as I go in to see her. Being at the hospital again just brings the whole nightmare back, and I'm so angry that once again it's a struggle to keep my temper. But the consultant can tell me nothing anyway. 'I'm sorry, but I don't know,' she says, holding her hands out. 'I can't explain, Mr Millthorpe. As you know, I saw your wife only four days before she died, and at that point she was having chemo and seemed fine. I was as shocked as you were,' she finishes.

Again, my anger flares. 'But all that *time*!' I persist. 'All that time when she was losing weight and you did *nothing*!'

I'm too upset now to continue. But, while I stand there shaking, the consultant looks back through the notes for the past six months. 'There's nothing here,' she says, back from when Angie saw the registrar in March, 'about you telling the doctor then about Angie's weight loss. But then in May,' she goes on, 'he's noted that Angie's weight has "stabilised", which contradicts what he put in the notes earlier.' She looks up at me. 'I'm so sorry, but there's nothing I can do. He doesn't work here any more; in fact, he's no longer in the UK, so I'm afraid I can't ask him about it.'

After the meeting, which has left me feeling even more frustrated, Lynne Handley does her best to calm me down.

'Ian,' she says, gently, as we walk back towards her office, 'it's possible Angie just died of her cancer. Perhaps you should just try to accept that.'

But I can't. I know everyone says I should. But I just can't.

On the way home, I stop at Angie's brother Neil's house, and tell him what the oncologist has told me. Which is essentially nothing, but Neil suggests that I leave Angie's medical notes with him. 'Let me take a look,' he says. 'See if I can see anything.'

Sure enough, a few days later, Neil telephones me, having now read Angie's notes. But he doesn't even mention her weight loss. 'Did you know our Angie was allergic to morphine?' he says instead.

'Of course,' I answer. 'They wouldn't have given her morphine. It's on her hospital records, too. The oncologist knows about it.'

Reece is in the room while I'm talking to Neil on the phone. 'Dad,' he says as soon as I've said goodbye to Neil, 'I'm sure I heard one of the nurses talking about morphine the night Mum died. I think that's what they gave her to help her pain.'

The next day I'm back at the hospital, but this time it's to get Angie's nursing records, which confirm that she *was* given morphine.

As soon as I'm back home I call the coroner again. There's still no result from the postmortem, but this is something new, and, when I explain that I have Angie's nursing records and that she was given morphine the night she died, he tells me there will now have to be an inquest.

'Which is like a court hearing,' he explains, 'so you'll have to do everything through a solicitor. Do you have a solicitor?'

I tell him I do. 'In that case, you need to put everything in his hands now, because everything from here on will need to be dealt with through him. And we'll let you know in due course about the date.'

All of this is a relief, and I'm pleased that I might get some peace of mind now – though it will change nothing. I put the phone down feeling empty inside. She's gone. And there's nothing that will bring her back.

The following week, Jake and Jade both turn eight, and I pull myself together enough to organise a party for them. I'm determined to make Angie proud of my efforts, so I decide to make their birthday cake myself.

I drop the children off that morning in a positive mood. It lightens my step a little to know I'm doing something to make Angie happy; even if she's not here physically, I sense her presence with me so intently.

Ella's excited. She loves helping with any sort of cooking, so I pull up a chair to the kitchen worktop so she can stand and work beside me, and I find a child's pinny in one of the kitchen drawers.

That done, she helps me cream the butter and sugar, then it's time to add the eggs. And, as Ella carefully passes them to me, one by one, I can't help but remember back to that day Angie got me back and got all that egg all down my face. It makes me smile. It's such a nice memory.

The mixture made, I transfer it into the cake tin to go in the oven, then it's time to make the buttercream filling.

'Yum,' I say, sticking in my finger once I'm finished. 'That's yummy, that, Ella,' I say, teasing her.

'Can I taste it, Dad?' she asks me, so I push the bowl across to her. 'Just a bit,' I say, 'not too much.' And she pokes her finger in.

'Yummy,' she agrees, nodding. 'Can I have some more?'

'Just a little more,' I tell her, because I don't want her making herself sick. 'Then it's time for us to go and do some hoovering.'

Ella loves hoovering. But it seems that today she has other ideas. I'm just finishing off the living room when I realise she's disappeared. Concerned that she might touch the hot oven door, I switch the vacuum cleaner off and go looking for her. Sure enough, she's back in the kitchen, but she's not near the oven. She's dragged the chair back up to the worktop, pulled the clingfilm off the bowl and is busily helping herself to more buttercream.

But she smiles Angie's smile, which means I can't even be cross with her. I'm going to have to watch that, I think.

The cake cool, slit in half and the buttercream in place, we set about making the icing. Once again, Ella 'helps', though I'm no better than she is, and the end result looks as if she did it on her own, I'm so bad. But I persevere, and the second coat turns out a little better, and, with time getting on, I set about decorating the top. It's a little bit ambitious, but I'm *feeling* ambitious, so, having rummaged in the drawers I pull out an icing bag and nozzle and, having fitted the latter and filled the former with icing, I set about carefully piping a scalloped edge all round the cake.

To my surprise, it really looks good. Good enough to impress Ella, too. 'Ooh, that's pretty, Dad!' she chirps, clapping her hands together. And she's right: it does, I couldn't be prouder. And when I add the pink and blue candles – eight for Jade and eight for Jake – it almost looks as if I could have bought it from a proper bakery.

'Lovely cake,' Ella says, as we give it pride of place on the party table. And, when Jake and Jade see it and are cooing with excitement, I feel a real sense of satisfaction in a job well done.

But I'm soon to come crashing down to earth again. It's only when I'm looking through my photo box a few weeks later that I pick up the notebook in which Angie wrote down the kids' birthdays and realise I've made a mistake. For all my baking success, I have still managed to fail her. I organised everything for 22 November. Jake and Jade's birthday is 21 November.

Doesn't matter that the twins didn't even realise my mistake. I've already let Angie down and I feel dreadful.

Chapter 22

I do better when it comes to Corey, who turns five two weeks later. I make another cake – though this time without Ella's help, as Glenn's looking after her – and get him the *Toy Story* figures he's been wanting so much. Time and time again, I wonder how I'd get by without my brother, who is a constant in my life now, and indispensable. Living so close, Glenn pops up to mind Ella while I take the kids to school each morning, and is on hand any time I have to go and run errands. As he doesn't work, he has all the time in the world for them, and they all love him to bits. He takes them to the park and out for walks, plays games with them and entertains them, and I constantly find myself thinking what a shame it is that he doesn't have any children of his own. I'm so grateful he's there for us.

And his calm presence in our lives means I'm coping day to day now at least. It's been such a shock, though, having to look after the kids without Angie. It's just so hard, in a million little ways. How do you cope with dressing one child while keeping an eye on the others; making dinner while they are clamouring for you to do something else for them; breaking up squabbles between two of them while trying to bath another? I've always known you need eyes in the back of your head with children, but now I feel I need them on either side as well.

But, despite this, Glenn's support allows me a glimmer of positivity about Christmas. And, though part of me would just like to cancel it for this year, I can't. I have the children to think about. I'm also reminded of how important it is that I face it, when I pop in to see Herbert a couple of weeks beforehand to find he's put up a few decorations. I didn't expect this. He never wanted any decorations up for Christmas. What with there being just him and Winnie and their being so elderly, he couldn't see the point. But Winnie loved Christmas every bit as much as Angie, so she'd nag him and nag him and she'd always get her way.

But she's gone now, and with her and Angie both having died so recently, never in a million years would I expect to walk into his house and find the little light-up Father Christmas in its usual place in the window, tinsel around all the pictures, and Christmas cards strung across the walls. I tell him so, and he gives me a little smile and shrugs.

'I just thought I'd put a few decorations up for Winnie, lad,' he says.

Angie was never any different from her mum, and our own Christmas tree's one we got in B&Q three years back. Angie saw it and she just had to have it, and that was that. I didn't see why at the time, since the one we had was only two years old and perfectly fine. But she just loved this one – it had holly berries and pine cones all over it – and she just went on about it till I caved in and bought it.

And now I'm so glad I did, because it feels so much *her* tree. And we all decorate it together, just as we always do, with the kids all taking turns to get the decorations out of the boxes, and me holding up the little ones so they can put them on the higher branches. Like every family, we have lots that the children made themselves, and, with so many kids in our house, that means *lots*. Finally, I lift Ella up above my shoulders, so she can be the one who puts the angel on the top. Not that we need one, I think as she puts it in position. We have our own angel, looking down and watching over us.

The tree up, I feel more confident I'll manage to get through it, because its presence in the living room makes me feel Angie's close to us. And at least Christmas gives me and the kids something else to focus on. Birthdays aside, it's been such a difficult few weeks, really, as the enormity of our loss begins to sink in, and the children try to adjust to carrying on without their mum.

I'm particularly worried about Jake, and so's Glenn, whom Jake's really close to. We've both noticed he seems to be fighting with his siblings constantly, and also, it turns out, at school.

One morning, about a month after Angie's death, I get a call from the school secretary. I'm in the middle of doing some washing when the house phone rings.

'I'm sorry to bother you, Mr Millthorpe,' she says. 'Only it's Jake. We're rather concerned about him.'

'Why?' I ask.

'Well, apparently, he got into a fight with another boy, stormed out of his classroom and then ran out of school. He's fine,' she quickly adds before I have a chance to worry about what's happened to him. 'He's back in school now, but he was in such a temper he almost got knocked down by a car running across the road when one of the teachers went after him.'

They ask me if I'll go in and have a quick word with the head when I come to pick them all up from school, and once I'm there they tell me how concerned they are about him, and how badly Angie's death has impacted on his behaviour. And it turns out to be the tip of the iceberg. I start getting calls from the school on a regular basis. Jake's been fighting. Jake's flared up with his teacher. Jake's fallen out with someone or other. And, though I keep going up and hearing about it, I don't know quite what to do about it. He's obviously reacting to losing his mum by lashing out, and I don't know how to begin to make it better. Do I come down hard on him when he's naughty, or do the exact opposite? If I'm finding it hard dealing with the practicalities of being a lone parent to so many children, I'm finding it so much harder knowing how to deal with the emotional stuff, trying to be both their mum and their dad at the same time. It was so simple when Angie was alive: I would always be the one who put his foot down when it was needed. But how can I do that now, when the children are already so upset? I find it almost impossible to tell them off.

But Teresa, the school nurse, has an idea. 'You know, Jake,' she says to him at yet another meeting following an incident. 'I think you would really benefit from some counselling,

Someone to talk to outside of the family, where you can let off steam.'

Jake looks anxious. He's clearly not that keen on having to talk to a stranger. But Teresa's quick to allay his fears. 'Jake, I'll be there too, if you'd like that,' she reassures him. 'And there's something else we could do together which I think you might enjoy. We could make a memory box, something to remind you of Mummy. We can put lots of special things in there: pictures of her, keepsakes, things she loved. How about that? Shall we do that together?'

Jake seems to like this idea better, and that's what they end up doing. Jake starts seeing the counsellor and at the same time he and Teresa make this beautiful box together. And it's clearly the best thing he could have done, because it allows him to feel close to Angie: almost every day he comes home from school and asks me for different photographs, and will sit and write her little notes that he can take in the next day. He's so excited when it's done and he brings it home to show me. It has little notes he's written to her that are on heart-shaped pieces of paper, and he's also made a dream catcher to hang up in his bedroom. It has a photo of his mum stuck in the middle of it, and little pieces of pipe hanging from it that jangle in the breeze.

The school are wonderful with Jade and Corey, too, and I'm so grateful for their care. Just before the end of term they have all three of them write letters to Angie, which they then fix to sky lanterns and light so they can fly away over the school field. It's such a lovely thing for them to do, and I can't thank them enough.

But, for all that, the end of term and Christmas can't come soon enough, even though part of me is dreading it. Although it's always been me who has bought and wrapped the majority of the presents, I know that 'doing' Christmas is going to be the biggest test of my training since Angie died. Despite everything Angie's taught me, I'm still floundering – particularly when it comes to getting the girls' presents – and I'm so incredibly busy in the days leading up to the big day that by the time Christmas Eve comes around I'm in awe. I can't quite believe that this is what Angie's been doing, every single Christmas, year after year after year.

But, to my surprise, the bit I have been most scared of – watching the children open their presents on Christmas morning, and opening mine from them – is actually okay. Though my heart aches for Angie and for all the Christmases she'll never have with them, I manage to get through that part without a single tear.

But you never know when grief is going to sneak up and overpower you. And that's what it feels like – as if you are powerless to stop it controlling your body. I'm in the middle of peeling the potatoes for our Christmas lunch when it happens.

Nat and Damon have arrived by now, with my eldest nephew, Adrian, Malc's son, and Nat's in the kitchen helping me at the time. I'm only vaguely aware that she must have slipped out and got the boys, because, seconds later, Damon and Adrian both have their arms around me. It takes a long time before my sobs subside, but I know they must. The children must not see me cry on Christmas Day. Angie would be furious.

*

After we've eaten our Christmas lunch, I take the five younger children down to the cemetery, the older boys already having visited her that morning. The sky is full of woolly, wintry clouds and there's snow on the ground, and Corey and Ella, red-cheeked from the cold, run ahead of us.

'Mummy! Mummy!' they both shout, their voices high and excited as we come to the part of the cemetery where Angie's grave is. Jake, Jade and Corey all made Christmas cards in school for her, and today they've brought them with them to give to her. The snow is thick on the ground because we had a fresh snowfall yesterday – it's been the snowiest Christmas I can remember for a while. And I wish Angie had lived to see it, because I know how much she would have loved it. She loved everything about Christmas, snow very much included, and I remember how she'd be peering endlessly out of the window and examining the clouds, any time a snowfall was forecast. 'Come on!' she'd tell the sky. 'Come on, snow, keep coming!' just as excitedly as any child would.

She'd love the snow on her grave today, I think, as we cross the crunchy ground and approach it. Here, where it's lying on all the holly wreaths and flowers, it's turned the grave into a cluster of pillowy, twinkling mounds. I kneel down to brush it away and reveal the flowers and berries once again, and, though I'm surprised they're holding up so well, in some ways I'm not. It feels only right that someone whose spirit was so alive should continue to breathe life into the place where she's at rest.

As I attend to the wreaths, and the little ones play in the

snow, the twins kneel down at the graveside with me, so they can talk to Angie. Jade chatters away, telling her mum about the new doll and pram Santa brought her, and Jake, who seems so much better now he's begun having his counselling, tells her all about how pleased he is with his new bike. Even though I know how much they miss her and that this period of joy is temporary, it's good to hear the happiness in their voices. Christmas has definitely given them all a boost. Connor got a bike from Santa too, but he is silent, and I completely understand that. He's reaching puberty now, an age where boys in particular are sensitive and emotional, and I know he'd rather keep his thoughts to himself than risk the embarrassment of breaking down in front of his younger siblings.

Being here with the children, I find it a huge effort of will not to cry too, but somehow I manage it, and am proud to have done so: it's my Christmas present to Angie. Today – Christmas Day – was her favourite day of the year. So no tears allowed, not from me.

We don't stay long. It's just so cold. Bitter cold, as it's been for days now. It's beautiful to look at, with the whole world coated in frost sparkles, but also the sort of cold that would have had Angie turning up the heating to the max. Angie was always cold, being so slim, even with the heating full on; and, as we leave the cemetery, a memory comes to mind of the two of us watching telly, and how we'd always sit the same way, I up at one end of the sofa, Angie stretched out along it.

'Lift your T-shirt up, Mill,' she'd say, 'so I can warm my feet up on your belly.'

I hate the thought of her being so cold. Hate that we're going home now, to our cosy house, and leaving her here in this cold, cold graveyard.

Every year of our marriage Angie and I went out on New Year's Eve. My brother Glenn never much likes going out, so he would babysit and we'd invariably go to the local pub with our huge family. And it's perhaps because of this, having just climbed the mountain that was Christmas, that I elect to stay in with Glenn this year, and be with my children, who need me there.

And we have a fine time – a better time than I could ever have imagined, in fact. We eat party food, watch TV and play board games with Glenn. And it's during the evening that we decide we will go on an adventure in a few weeks, make our first trip of the year to Thornwick – just for the day – and, while we're there, book a summer holiday too.

Thornwick opens for the season in early March, and, by the time we get to it, I'm glad. It's been hanging over me a bit, even though the kids have been so excited, because I know making the journey there will be a huge hurdle to jump. It was Angie's favourite place in all the world and I will see her round every corner; there's not an inch of the place that won't stir up memories. And, as I expect, even though the kids are really hyper when we set off (or perhaps because of that), as I drive the hire car along the familiar route without her I feel a sense of dread about how I'll cope.

It's a beautiful day. A little chilly still, but sunny, and it's definitely encouraged everyone out. It's almost as busy as you'd expect in high summer, the car park almost full and people everywhere. We go rock-pooling first, clambering around and over the rocks at the cliff base, looking for crabs and fish and starfish. And it doesn't take long till Jake finds a crab – a big one. Well, not *that* big, not from where I'm standing, but by the hullabaloo going on you'd think it was a monster. 'Dad! *Daaad!*' he yells, the offending animal firmly clamped around his finger. 'Dad! Get it off me! *Oww!* Get it *off* me, Dad! *Help!*'

I'm laughing so hard as I pick my way across to rescue him from its clutches that I almost slip on the rocks and get a soaking. And it's a tiddly little thing – probably glad to be back in the water and away from Jake's screeching. We're all of us in fits of laughter now, and it feels really good.

The other thing we do when we're rock-pooling is gather winkles, which can be found in huge quantities, stuck to the sides of the rocks. I get my plastic bag out – I always have one, for just this purpose – and get an impressive haul to take home to my brother, Terry, who'll boil them up, then he and Diane will pull them out with a pin and eat them.

We all love winkles, so gathering them when we're at Thornwick and out rock-pooling is a family tradition; the kids have been feasting on them on holiday for years. And, as the kids pop them one by one into my plastic bag, I'm reminded of the time I gave Angie a live one, when she thought it was one of the ones I'd already cooked. 'Oh, Mill!' she said, as she poked it and it retracted back into its shell. 'Yuck! You so-and-so. I should have known you were up to something!' And then she threw it at me. The memory still makes me smile.

After we've been rock-pooling, everyone wants to go into the park itself. They always do, because they all love the play area. 'Daddy, Daddy!' They're all nagging me, talking over each other as usual. 'Can we go in the park?' 'Can we go in the play area?' 'Can we go on all the amusements?'

I have enough coins in my pocket to keep everyone happy, and I'm actually happy myself to take a walk around the park because it's nice to see familiar faces – we've been coming so long that lots of the staff know us – and because, while we're there, we do what we've often done over the years: take a look at all the caravans that are up for sale. It's only ever been a pipe dream, especially since I was invalided out of mining, but, year on year, we'd pop along to the sales office on the site and borrow the keys so we could look around a few. 'One day,' Angie would always say, 'one day, Mill, we'll have one.' And the kids would join in, then. 'Please, Daddy, please!'

Then and there I decide that, one day, we will.

We finish up with a stroll around Bridlington. Coming to Bridlington while we're up here is always part of any trip to Thornwick. It's quite a posh seaside place, Bridlington, with a grand Victorian seafront, a harbour with lots of boats in, a funfair and a big sandy beach. You can also go on boat rides out of Bridlington harbour, one of which is on a big pirate ship. There's also some kiddy bumper boats with petrol engines in them, and today I hire two – one for me, Jade, Corey and Ella and the other for Connor and Jake. I let the kids steer, as they always do, and enjoy the sound of them all laughing as they steer the boats into each other again and again, imagining Angie looking down and loving it too.

Once we're done on the front, I tell the children they can all choose a toy each. They're all pleased to hear this and we start looking in all the little seaside shops in the arcades, though, as ever, there's only one thing that interests Connor and Jake – the prospect of getting a new game for the Xbox. And, of course, once we get one, they want to go straight home to play on it. But we don't linger, anyway, as we have one place left to go.

The toys chosen, we set off back up to the cliff top. It was being up here, with the stunning views of the cliffs, that Angie loved best. It was one of her favourite spots in the world. We call in the café and get teas for me and Connor, and cola for the younger ones, and it's while we're in there that I remember what it is I want to do.

There's a row of benches outside the café, all of them bearing brass plaques, in memory of loved ones who've died. Angie always loved reading them, and always commented on what a nice idea they were, so it's always been on my mind that I should get one done for her.

'That's a brilliant idea, Dad,' Jade says excitedly, as I tell her what I'm planning to do. We even choose the bench. There are so many plaques that there are few spaces left for new ones, but we find one on a bench that the kids agree has the best view.

We pop back into the café then, to ask if they know where we can get one made for Angie, and, since we're here, one in memory of my mum and dad too, from me and my brothers and sister.

'Oh, it's my husband who makes those,' the lady on the till tells me. 'I just need you to write down where you want it and exactly what you want it to say.

I put, 'In loving memory of my beautiful wife, Angela Rose Millthorpe, died 19/10/10. I miss you more and more each passing day. All my love, Mill xxx.' And, as we head for home, I make myself another promise: that one day, when I can afford it, I'll buy her a bench of her very own.

Chapter 23

You'd be a fool to think coming to terms with losing someone dear to you would be easy, and as the weeks roll on, and our lives begin to find a new rhythm, Angie's absence feels every bit as hard to bear still.

And it shows itself in different ways with the different children. Jake's calmer now, seems to have got some of his energy (not to mention mischievousness) back, but now it's Connor who's causing me concern. It's easy to forget that, in the middle of everything, he's going through his first year in high school, which is a massive thing in itself, and has made everything doubly stressful.

The signs are all there. He starts inventing spurious illnesses on school mornings, and telling me he doesn't want to go to school. It takes a while to coax out of him what's really troubling him, but he eventually confesses that boys have been name-calling, and that someone's even threatened to beat him up after school.

I'm sickened and disgusted – how could anyone be so horrible to a child going through what he is? So I immediately ring the school and make an appointment to see the headmaster. He's mortified, understandably, when I go in to see him, and promises he'll speak to the parents of the boys involved.

'I hope so,' I tell him, 'because, if you don't, I will.' It's all I can do not to do just that anyway.

But, whatever the head has or hasn't done, the bullying doesn't stop. Just a few weeks later, I get a phone call from him again. He's got Connor in his office, clearly very upset. I can tell that from how he is when he speaks to me on the phone.

'What's been going on?' I ask him. And in a broken voice he tells me that one boy in particular just keeps chanting this song at him.

'What song?' I ask him.

Connor can hardly speak for sobbing. 'It goes, "Where's your mamma gone?",' he eventually tells me.

I put the phone down furious. I am almost speechless at such cruelty.

Over the next few days, however, Connor's problems are, thankfully, resolved. Once the parents of the boys are notified about what happened, I even have my faith in human nature restored. Connor comes home from school a couple of days later with a question.

'Dad,' he says. 'You know Jack? Jack who was singing that song to me?'

'Yes,' I say. I could hardly forget.

'Well,' he says, 'it's just that he's been over an' said he's sorry, and we've made friends now an' he's coming round and calling for me later an' he wants me to tell you he's really sorry for what he did an' that it won't happen again.'

I nod, as Connor gets his breath back after his little speech. I'm still sceptical: why would you want to make friends with someone who's just been so unkind to you? I hope he's not just being wound up again. But I must take him at his word. I can hear Angie telling me that's the right way. He clearly wants to be friends with this boy, and who am I to come between them?

'That's fine,' I say. 'If you've accepted his apology then so do I, son.'

Sure enough, later on, there's a knock at the front door, and I open it to see a very nervous-looking boy standing on the doorstep.

'I'm really sorry, Mr Millthorpe,' he says, 'for calling Connor names at school. We've made friends now so is it okay for me to be mates with him again?'

I look sternly at him, but, actually, I'm impressed at his courage. And I'm impressed by his politeness as well. 'Course you can,' I say, smiling. 'Come on in, lad.'

Connor and he remain firm friends to this day.

Domestically, too, I seem to be coping. Still smarting from my lapse over Jake and Jade's party, I am determined to remember my oldest boys' birthdays, which all fall around the end of March and beginning of April. And I do. I give the oldest two money, so they can treat themselves, and for Reece, who is busy starting up his own business with his friend Benji, I splash out on a laptop, which I know he really needs.

But it's the little things that still test me every day. Alone, I can still no longer pop anywhere to do anything. Whereas once I could jump in the car and run errands – get something for Herbert, grab some shopping, see one of my brothers – suddenly, if none of the older ones are around, I'm marooned. If I want to do anything, go anywhere, get anything done, I have to take all the kids with me. This annoys and inconveniences them every bit as much as it does me, particularly if they're having fun doing something else.

I am also not immune from making stupid mistakes. Just before Easter I buy Jade a new pair of red jeans, and, when she asks me to wash them one Saturday night, just before bedtime, I duly pop them in the washing machine ready for the next day. The next afternoon, of course, having forgotten that they're in there, I do a white wash in readiness for school. In go all the pristine white polo shirts, ready. And out they all come, nice and pink. Which is no way to send the kids in – particularly the boys – so they all get an unscheduled Monday morning off, and I have to shell out for a load of new ones.

I also have the issue of being a father to two daughters, which throws up difficult situations all the time. On our March trip to Thornwick, for instance, when Ella wanted to go to the toilet, I obviously had no choice but to take her in the Gents. Or, rather, try to – as soon as I did she kicked up merry hell. 'I'm not going in there, Daddy!' she wailed. 'That's the misters' one! I need the other one!' And, try as I might to calm her down and take her in, she was having none of it.

It was Jade who came to the rescue, even though she seemed too young herself to be doing it. 'I'll take her into the Ladies, Dad,' she said. 'We'll be all right.' Which meant an anxious wait outside for me while Jade got Ella sorted, but what else was I to do?

But the weeks stack up, and with each one, domestically, it gets easier. And, before we know it, it's May and our holiday is soon due.

There's one last grim thing I have to deal with before that day comes, however, and it's to travel to Sheffield on 3 May to attend the inquest into Angie's death. I've never been into a court, but I have an image of what they look like, from watching the television, and the Medico-Legal Centre in Sheffield looks like that. There's a raised platform for the coroner, who sits behind a desk, and a witness stand just to the side. Everyone else sits facing them, in seats like those you'd see in a cinema, each row raised slightly higher than the one in front of it.

Several members of the family come with me: Reece, Malc and Eileen, and our Karen, as well as Angie's brother Neil, and Diane. And I'm grateful to have them there because it's a long emotional day, starting at ten in the morning, and not finishing till three. Witness after witness takes the stand, from the experts who are brought in, to the nurse who looked after Angie the night she died. She can't recall the exact sequence of events that night clearly, but, when Angie's blood pressure dipped so low at 8 p.m., can't believe she wouldn't have bleeped the doctor straightaway.

There's lots of discussion about the issue of Angie being allergic to codeine and tramadol, but, though it's obvious to me that she had an adverse reaction to those kinds of drugs, the coroner's verdict doesn't differ from what was first written on the death certificate. Once again, he records the cause of death as being due to disseminated malignancy, i.e. the cancer that had spread throughout Angie's body. There is apparently no evidence of a major bleed due to the burst ulcer Angie suffered that morning, but neither is there evidence of anaphylaxis, apparently (a severe allergic reaction to having been given morphine).

It *is* noted that, however sketchy the recollection of the nurse on duty, when, at 8 p.m., Angie's blood pressure was very low, no doctor attended till her cardiac arrest at 9 p.m. But this isn't key, the coroner explains, saying that, even if a doctor *had* attended sooner, it wouldn't have made a difference to the outcome.

I sit there and listen to all this, digesting what he's saying and trying to reconcile myself to it. But it's so hard to, and I think perhaps now I never will, because, whatever I'm hearing about the details of what did or didn't happen, the sense of 'what if?' lingers: I still can't quite accept that she never got that chance.

As we all head home that day, another feeling weighs heavily on me. Guilt. Guilt that I ever took Angie into hospital that day. What if I hadn't taken her? What if I'd turned around at the roundabout and taken her home again? Would she still be here with us today? There's no question that the outcome was always going to be this one, but it tortures me to think that she might have had longer, might have enjoyed her children for just a few more precious months, and – who knows? – maybe even years.

Thinking of the children and what they've lost gives me a rush of immense sadness – and self-pity, too, much as I know I mustn't feel that way. But, even as I think that, I feel Angie's presence beside me, feel her voice in my ear, saying, 'No, Mill!' I remember the day we were told that her cancer was terminal, and how bravely and stoically she accepted her fate. 'What's the point in worrying,' she consoled me when I was completely inconsolable, 'about something you can do absolutely *nothing* about?'

Of all the lessons I've learnt from my wise, courageous wife, perhaps this is the one I need most now.

Chapter 24

Angie never dwelt on the past. If there's one thing that always brings my wonderful wife to mind, it's when I hear people going on about something that's already happened. Something they can do nothing about.

'What's done is done,' Angie always used to say. It was a maxim she used often about little things – she was never one to cry over spilt milk – and about the big things as well. 'We can't alter the past,' she'd always remind me, 'but we can change the future.'

It's something I've had to keep reminding myself of while living through what have been the most terrible few months of my life. And, largely, it's worked. I'm trying to do things her way. Getting on, making the best of it, not wasting time wishing things had been different. And more and more I find I'm inclining towards Angie's way of thinking, having decided that, however much I wish she'd stayed longer, being the lucky man who got to have such an incredible woman, I've not been dealt a bad hand after all. In fact, more and more I realise I was actually dealt four aces.

And if my resolve weakens, or if I have a bad day – which

I do, and do expect to – I have this powerful sense that she's not so far away.

I'm doing some housework one such day, vacuuming the living room while the kids are in school, when I stop and turn the hoover off, just to look at her picture – the one that Neil and Diane had framed for me and gave me for Christmas.

'God, I miss you, love,' I tell her. 'God, how I wish you were still here with us.'

And with that – almost in the exact instant I say those words to her – the picture falls off the wall and lands right on top of my stockinged feet. And as I'm hopping around the room in agony, I swear I can hear her laughing.

Even more curiously, when I go to put it back, I find the hook on the back of the picture is still in place, as is the one on the wall. 'Don't worry, Mill,' I imagine Angie saying. 'I'm still here.'

Spooky. Very spooky. But nice.

There's no getting away from it – I'm dreading it. But in May 2011, just as Angie asked me to in her list, I finally take the children to Thornwick Bay for their first family holiday without her. It's even harder than I thought it would be, as well. Neil and Diane were planning on coming, which would have made the whole thing so much more bearable, but in the end they have to pull out, right at the last minute, because their little granddaughter Harri is poorly.

It's just the five youngest children coming with me on this occasion again, because Reece is hard at work with his and

Benji's fledgling business, which is beginning to build up very promisingly. I know I'll miss having him there, as he's such a support to me. But I'm so proud of him – so proud of all my grown-up boys, making such a go of their lives, in the midst of such a tragedy.

I hire another people carrier, and the older children are wonderful in helping with all the packing. Already I can see Jade's becoming quite the little mum, taking care of Ella in a way that seems to be becoming automatic.

'Dad, don't forget this!' she says, passing me Ella's favourite doll. 'And did you remember to pack the sunblock for Ella?' She turns to Ella herself then. 'Now,' she says, 'do you need to go to the toilet before we leave? It'll be a long time before you'll have a chance to go again.'

Which makes me smile, but it's fleeting, because, as soon as we set off, it feels every bit as bad as I expected. Every aspect of the journey is so familiar, so predictable, that Angie's absence screams out at me all the way there. Connor's there beside me in the front, seeming so grown up now that it breaks my heart to look at him. I'm so relieved that he seems so much happier at school now. He's at such a vulnerable age, and losing his mum has hit him hard. But Angie's ghost seems to sit beside us too. I remember the way she'd unwrap sweets to give to me, take the top off a bottle of pop for me. Such little things. But they really are the big things when they've gone.

But, once we get there, the magic of the place seems to do its work on me and, as we unload the car in the warm sunshine and get all our belongings unpacked in the chalet, I begin to replace some of the constant gnawing pain with happy memories of the many laughs we've shared here. And will have again, I think, because that's what we came for. That was why Angie made me promise we wouldn't stop.

Once we're unpacked, and Connor and I have sat and had a cup of tea, we have an important first job to attend to. We pile back into the car, leave the park, and take the familiar narrow lane that winds up to the cliff-top café.

As soon as we see the bench with Angie's plaque on, it lifts all our spirits. The plaque is new and shiny, and when we all sit down, as Angie used to, the view is perfect, looking out over the towering white cliffs, and the caves that we've explored so many times over the years. I swear I can feel her presence here with us.

'We gotta get some flowers, Dad!' Connor says, looking at the benches around us, which all seem to be accessorised with floral tributes of some kind, either laid beside them or tied on with string.

'Yes, flowers!' agrees Jade, tugging at my arm. 'Mum needs some flowers!' She seems happy. It's so good to see her smiling.

I find myself smiling, too. There is almost a note of celebration in the air, and, wanting to hang on to it, I decide we should drive into nearby Bridlington and get some flowers to put on Angie's bench then and there.

The kids argue about what to get for most of the short journey there, but, by the time we've parked up and found a florist, we're all in agreement. We get a big bunch of roses for Angie from me, and five single red roses, one for each child.

And when we get back we place them all by the side of her bench.

'There,' says Jade. 'Mum'll love all those, won't she? Because red was her favourite colour, weren't it, Dad? I bet she's looking down from Heaven and smiling about all these flowers.'

There's a short silence, while we all look at the roses. And we do smile.

'My mum was *always* smiling,' Jade says firmly.

The weather is kind to us at Thornwick, as it so often is, and we spend most of our time on the beach. We go rock-pooling again, and build elaborate sandcastles, just as we always would when Angie was here too. We play ball games and paddle (it's not quite warm enough for swimming), and I realise I'm managing to do both the dad things *and* the mum things; I am coping. The children seem to be having fun and their joy is infectious – both a relief and a shot in the arm for me.

And we are obviously something of a novelty down on the beach. Time and again, while we're down there, people come over and talk to us, and want to know how I manage on my own with so many kids. And, when I tell them about Angie, everyone's always so kind, telling me how proud I should be of such lovely children, and how well I'm bringing them up.

'Can you hear that?' I keep saying to myself, knowing Angie's listening. 'Are you proud of me, love?' And I like to think she is.

On the third day at Thornwick, I take the kids back to Bridlington. There's a shop there that sells all the usual beachy trinkets, and we decide to see if we can find a little ornament to put under Angie's headstone back home, to add to the ever-growing collection.

Angie's Gates of Heaven headstone was laid at the end of January, and since then we've been bringing her little gifts. There are two seals – because Angie always loved seals. One's from the children and one's from Neil and Diane, who also bought the snow globe with her picture in. There's also a silver picture frame in the shape of two rings that has photos of Angie and me in them, and a small porcelain angel I found for her.

We're just looking in the window to see what they have, when an elderly lady starts chatting to the kids.

'What wonderful children you have,' she says, turning to me. Then she turns to Jade. 'Are you waiting for your mum?'

'My mummy died,' Jade explains. 'We're going to buy a new ornament for her grave.'

The children all chime in then, all wanting to tell her about Angie. 'She's got a bench,' Connor says proudly. 'And Dad got them to make a plaque for it.'

'And it says, "We miss you",' Jake chips in. 'And we already bought some flowers for it. Roses.'

'Flowers,' Ella confirms. 'Flowers for Mummy.'

'She loved dachshund dogs and seals,' Jade tells the lady, 'so that's what we're looking for.'

And as I look on I begin to feel sorry for the poor woman. Her eyes are now brimming with unshed tears.

'Oh, I'm so sorry,' she says, turning to look at me. 'So, so sorry.'

Her friend comes out of the shop then, and she hugs me goodbye. 'They are *lovely*,' she whispers. 'You are doing such a great job with them. I bet your wife's looking down at you and bursting with pride.'

But the best moment comes a while later, back in the chalet. We always liked to book chalet 10 when we visited, one with a view of the play area, so we could keep an eye on the kids, and the patio door with a panoramic view over the surrounding fields. Standing looking out there now, I feel Angie's presence keenly.

But I'm calm – and something else, besides: accepting. This is my life now, and I'm determined to live it the way she wanted. To devote all my energies to the children she blessed me with, so that when I fetch up in Heaven she won't give me grief. That she'll welcome me with open arms, and tell me I've done her proud. Just as her children, I reckon, are doing her proud already. Six months in and I just know they'll be okay.

I go into the kitchen to make a start on tea. Jake and Jade have walked the dogs, the boys have gone to let off steam in the play area and Jade and Ella are playing quietly together in the bedroom. Or, rather, *were* playing quietly. I'm just rustling up the ham salad when the pair of them appear in the kitchen doorway, Jade leading Ella in to be inspected.

I've noticed this lately. How Jade's become this proper little mum to Ella. She watches everything I do these days, and she's so keen to learn. There've been that many times lately when the pair of them have gone upstairs and, when they've come down again, Ella's had the whole makeover treatment:

completely different set of clothes, completely different hair-style. And, though it hurts to think that Angie's missing something so sweet to witness, I'm also comforted by seeing what a lovely bond my girls have, and will hopefully always have, particularly since they don't have a mummy. Angie was so right. It's brilliant she had a second daughter.

Jade's got a grin on her face as wide as anything. 'Dad,' she says excitedly, as I wipe my hands. 'Look!'

She spins Ella round so I can see what she's been up to.

'See, Dad!' she says, beaming. 'Aren't I clever?'

And she is. As I say, she's a great little learner. She's styled Ella's hair into a perfect French plait, and, in my head at least, I'm looking up, hoping Angie can see it too. See that things are working out – see that things *will* work out. See that we're managing. That we're all doing it *her* way.

But I don't need to lift my eyes because I *know* Angie's there.

See that, love? I think, proudly.

Because I taught her.

Epilogue

Raising our children single-handed makes me realise why Angie was always smiling, despite having to put so much work into it. I know, because all the hard work I now do to bring them up Angie's way is far outweighed by the love and enjoyment they give me in return.

Our big lads are all men now, and I know how proud she'd be of the three of them. Ryan's got a lovely girlfriend, whom he's living with over in Cudworth, and is working hard for a new firm who've just set up there; and Damon – who's also with a new girlfriend – is still living and working in Grimethorpe.

Natalie's made a new start, in Sutton-on-Sea, but there'll never be a time we don't see her as family. She and Angie were so close, and she was a tower of strength to me and the kids at a terrible time. She's a brilliant mum to little Warren, and brings him down to see all the children regularly.

Reece's kitchen-fitting business is beginning to get established now and, despite the recession, he and his partner Benji are doing well. He's still with Sophie, who works at Next – and is still so wonderful with all the children – and they're hoping to get married one day. But there's no rush, and I suspect it's because I look after him too well at home – plus, my cooking's a lot better than Sophie's . . .

As for the younger ones, well, they're all doing their mum proud, and all have their individual personalities. Connor's the quiet one. He's such a helpful lad, always willing to give me a hand around the house and out in the garden. And, when he's got some time off from all the chores, he likes playing football and riding his bike best, and when he leaves school he'd like to go and work with Reece.

Jake's our giggler. Just like his mum, he's always laughing, and when he starts he can never stop. He's also very ticklish – he's not grown out of that, yet, Angie! – so, when I'm bathing him, washing under his arms is an impossible task. Like Connor, he's always happy playing football or riding his bike, and he's also hyper – full of energy – and I'm beginning to see why Angie told me how important it is to be firm with him. Give in to Jake and the next time he asks for something, and I say no, I have a screaming do on my hands!

Jade's our carer, so like her mum in so many ways. She gives Ella so much love, always ready with hugs and kisses, and loves dressing her up and messing with her hair. Give Jade a doll and a pram and she's happy. She does really well at school – she loves it. She also likes drawing, and is very good at it, too. Jade's always helpful, happy to do housework and help with baking. When she grows up she wants to be a teacher.

Corey's the cheeky one, very, very mischievous. But he'll have to grow out of it eventually, because when he grows up he wants to be a policeman. He and Ella are very close, but they don't much like having to share me. And Corey's the jealous one: if I give anything to Ella he wants it – even if it's a doll. I expect he'll grow out of that as well.

Ella's a mini-Jade: she loves her kisses and cuddles and loves playing with her dolls in the way Jade plays with hers: always dressing them up and pushing them round the garden in her pram. Ella loves to dance. She's always standing in front of the telly if there's a pop song on, making us all laugh when she cheekily wiggles her bum. So far, Ella most wants to be a nurse.

I see so much of Angie in the kids – particularly the girls, who are so like her. I have no doubt in my mind that they'll make great mothers to their own children, because I see her mothering instinct in them all the time. It's just so sad that this horrible disease robbed them of their own mother. But there's one thing cancer could never do. It could never take away the love we feel for Angie. We love her more and more with every passing day. And cancer could never take Angie out of our lives, either. We remember her with a smile every day.

My life now revolves around the children. It's now been over two years since Angie passed away and my grief is as raw today as it was the day she died. I visit her grave daily and at weekends I take all the kids, and before Ella leaves her mother's grave she always kisses the photo of Angie on the headstone and waves goodbye, saying, 'See ya later, Mummy!' And I'm lucky. It's through Ella that I still see Angie's amazing smile every day – she was fortunate to inherit that from her mum.

I'm raising the children the way Angie showed me to – the best way, Mum's way. I could never replace her, and I know I will never try to. She may be gone, but she's still with us, and I want to do her proud, so in my twilight years I can look back and <u>feel</u> proud as well. Not only that, I want to do it because I always have this picture of her, standing at the Pearly Gates, hands on hips, just as she used to, with a cross look on her face, saying, 'Right, Mill! Now you're for it!'

My Angie was a gem. And I take great comfort in knowing that, when the time comes, I'll leave this world with a smile on my face, because I'll be laid to rest with the woman I love so much – together forever with my childhood sweetheart.

Rest in peace, my beautiful Angie. And thank you for choosing me to share your amazing life with. Till we meet again,

All my love,
Mill x
December 2012

Dear Mum ...

This is the point at which I let others express their love for Angie in their own words, beginning with letters from our children.

To mummy,
You were the best mummy in all the world, you were a funny mummy. and i love you loads and loads, you always tickled me and made me laugh. love you forever and ever mummy.
Corey Ian

To mummy, love you mummy, you made me laugh, and gave me lots and lots of kisses, and i see you shining in the sky at night, because you're an angel now and daddy shows me your special star. you are the best mummy in the whole world,
Loves hugs and kisses, Ella Rose

To mum,
I love you so much, we still have fun when we go on holiday and dad always takes us on the boats and tells us lots of jokes and makes us laugh and he always takes us to the water park and we always feed the ducks like you did, and I always work hard at school like you told me to. And when we go on holiday we always look at your plaque and put flowers on it. We will always remember your

lovely face and your giggles. And I always laugh when you used to call me Danny long legs instead of Jake. You always gave us lots of hugs and kisses and when I kiss dad I give him one for you too. And my dad always buys us lots of toys and he's going to buy me a guitar like his and learn me to play some songs. And my dad told me you used to like feraro roshes and you used to hide them so he didn't pinch them. We will never forget your laugh and smile. And when you went on holiday with us you always took us on all the rides, and your favourite meal when you were on holiday were fish and chips and dough nuts. You and my dad are the best couple in all the world.

Love you mummy, Jake xxx

To mummy,

I will always love you and when daddy gets old like granddad we will take care of him. we still have lots of fun with dad when we go on the beach and he always takes us on the boats and on all the rides at the fair, when we go on holiday we go to the cafe and look at your plaque, When daddy is not busy he always takes us to the water park and we always feed the ducks for you. We still have lots of fun. Dad gave us your bedroom for me and Ella to share. When I kiss daddy I give him one for you too. I take care of your sausage dog that dad bought you for Christmas. And I sometimes help daddy to dress Ella for school. We have lots of pictures of you on the walls and I always do my homework like you told me to and work hard at school and at the queens jubilee party at school I won first prize for my dress that daddy bought me.

Lots of kisses, love you forever mummy, Jade xx

To mum,

I wish you were still with us mum, I love you so much, I miss hearing your funny laugh, you always made me laugh, we have pictures of you on every wall and dad has you tattooed on his chest, I work hard at school like you said, and we still go on lots of holidays and have lots of fun, I always help dad.

Love you mum Connor xxx

To mum,

I miss you so much mum, I miss all the laughs we had together, but I'll never forget the way you dealt with your illness in the last few years of your life, nothing seemed to get you down – not even this horrible disease cancer could wipe that smile from your face, you laughed till the very end, you had the courage of a gladiator Mum. Not only a wonderful caring loving mother, but a brave one too, I'm so proud to have had a mother like you, you always told me to try to do something with my life, well I've took your advice mum, and now I have set up my own business, I hope to do you proud mum, like you did us, I'll never forget you , you were SIMPLY THE BEST,

ALL MY LOVE, REECE, XXX

Mam, your life was full of loving deeds,
    forever thoughtful of our special needs,
    today, tomorrow, my whole life through,
    I will always love and cherish you.
    All my love Damon xx

To my wonderful mother,
    How proud I feel to have had a mother like you, you
were one in a million mam, I will never forget that
wonderful laugh of yours, There was never a dull
moment in our house with you around, I just wish you
could have been with us to see my first child Isaac,
you're always in my thoughts mam, and always will be,
love you forever,
    Ryan xx

Dear Angie . . .
    What can you say about a sister like our Angie?
    She was the best sister a brother could wish for. She
was kind, happy, and never had a bad word to say about
anyone. In fact, she was just like the Bruno Mars song,
Amazing just the way she was. I suppose one of the
things everyone will remember her for is her laugh, I can
remember the first day I took my girlfriend, now wife
Diane home to meet the family for the first time, as I
walked down the garden path with Diane our Angie was
stood in the upstairs window, laughing out LOUD. Diane

looked at me and said who's that? I just smiled at Diane and said that's our Angie, she's mad.

But, no doubt she'll still be looking down on us now still having a good laugh.

When our Angie was taken from us it broke my heart in two. I miss her loads.

I will always love you Angie,

From Brother Neil. Xxx

The way I'll always remember my beautiful Daughter Angela Rose. We spent so many happy times together sharing hours of fun, and you enriched the years for me with everything you've done,

Of all the Daughters in this world you were one in a million I would say, and there couldn't be more happiness in the 48 years you gave me.

So wherever you are in heaven, I hope you're still laughing and ear pulling with your mum Winnie.

God bless you both, and give each other a cuddle and a kiss from me.

All my eternal love, Dad xx

To Angie,

There's not a day goes by that I don't think of you, I miss you more with each passing day, This terrible disease took away not only my wonderful future mother in law, but my best friend too, we shared some wonderful happy times together, When the time comes for me to have children of my own, I won't let them forget what an amazing woman their nan nan Angie was.

R.I.P. Angie,

love Sophie xx

Angie was a great and beautiful young woman, but she was a greater wife, mother, and sister in law. Her children were her whole life together with her husband. Her laugh was just great, it was so infectious, you just knew it was Angie when you heard it. She is so sadly missed, but our loss is heaven's gain. All our love,

Malc and Eileen xx

I miss my sister Angie so much, she was like a best friend to me. Always laughing even though she was so ill. Angie lived for her children, they were her whole world. I'd call in to see her weekly and she'd always make me a coffee and then fill me in on all the latest gossip from near and far. The days come and go, but the pain and emptiness remain. I will never forget you Angie.

All my love, Wendy xx

Our Angie was the happiest person I've ever met, she was always laughing even when things weren't funny. No one could ever be sad with our Angie around, Angie hated seeing anyone feeling down. I can still hear her laugh as though it was only yesterday. Our Angie will always be in our hearts, we will cherish every precious moment we spent with her.

Love you always Angie,

Jonathan, Joni and children xxx

I've known Angie from her being a little girl who lived next door to me, and watched her grow into a wonderful wife and mother. Who would have guessed we would marry two brothers?

Angie lived her life for her family, but life can be so cruel, sometimes you are dealt bad cards, sadly Angie was. But she put more into life than most, and dealt with whatever life threw at her with great courage and dignity.

Angie loved children, and will always be remembered for having a big family. But i think her family will remember her for her infectious laugh.

RIP Angie,

from Lynn and Barry

To my sister Angie, You were the most beautiful, caring and loving sister anyone could wish for, and so brave to the very end. I will never forget you, you will always be in our hearts for ever. We think of all the wonderful holidays we had together at Rhyl, Flamborough, and Benidorm and all the fun and laughter we shared together. Me and Terry will always have a piece of our hearts missing, that piece Angie is you.

Love you always Angie,

Diane, Terry, Carina and Kane

When I was asked would I like to write a few words about Angie I felt very honoured and proud to be asked. But a few words would never be enough to write about this amazing lady.

Angie will have been many things to many people, but it was apparent her role in life was to be a wife and a mother to her husband Ian and her 8 children, she spoke of them in a whisper full of love and she showed in her eyes to me the fear she really felt. I am a mother of 4 and over the course of 2 years I have never met anyone so devoted to their family.

Angie had presence that few people have, she did not need to be angry or raise her voice to get your attention, she just had to walk in the room and smile. One day in particular when they both came to see me I was worried, concerned what the visit was about. Angie came in the room with Ian and sat down. I thought she looked beautiful and really well. I said 'Angie, you look well and your hair looks fabulous.' She proceeded to whip off her wig. I was so shocked I didn't have a clue. I looked at her, not knowing how to react, trying to be professional, when I saw her lips curl and a smile appear, then laughter, I laughed too, followed by Ian. How amazing that she was able to fetch humour into such a tense and difficult meeting. But that was Angie, she knew how hard it was for Ian and in her way she tried to lighten the mood to protect him.

One of the visits I had with Angie and Ian prior to an appointment with the oncologist, Angie started to tell me that this was the last week she would have her own teeth, I looked a bit flabbergasted, didn't really understand what she meant. I looked at Ian and Angie and said what do you mean? She explained she was trying a new medication, but as one of her teeth was loose, they felt the gum would not be able to heal, therefore to be involved in the trial she would have to have all her teeth removed. I was horrified, I asked her how she could be so brave, and very quietly she said I have to do anything that will let me be with my family a bit longer. She smiled at me and I looked back at Ian who was visibly upset. Angie just said "oh it's okay my false teeth will be perfect, I'll have a film star smile!" I sat in awe of this brave lady that accepted anything that was thrown at her, I was amazed by her bravery and I still am.

Lynne Handley
PALS representative

Angie was one of my best friends
    when I think of you, I remember the good times we shared
    the caravan holiday to golden sands Mablethorpe with
my family,
    the holiday to Rhyl in Wales with your family.

the blackpool day trip we dressed as twins.
the same clothes we used to wear
the high Sacha shoes we couldn't walk in.
the smile you always had
the famous laugh
the day you told me at Willowgarth high school you
fancied Milly
and I had to ask him if he would meet you
the day he said yes your smile lit up.
the chalking on the valley walls, and on the walls in the
pavilion that said ANGIE + MILLY TOGETHER 4 EVER
Memories I will never forget of a great friend
Love Angie (Henstock) xx

To Angie, Your love, your smile, your laugh I will always
remember.
You were always so tender,
Your strength was never failing,
Most of all your undying love for your family was
always true. Tenderly I treasure the past and memories
that will always last.
Angie was a gift sent from heaven who shared her love
and strength with everyone she touched.
I miss you, but the legacy you left lives on in your
children.
Teresa Clark,
Nursery nurse,
Milefield Primary School.

Angie was such a loving and gentle woman, Her wonderful personality touched so many lives, especially ours, Her smile could light up a room. I remember Angie coming to our house with Ian to my husband's 80th birthday party, even though she had just completed her first course of chemotherapy her laughter filled the house and made us all laugh with her. She never dwelled on her illness, she just seemed to make the very best of the time she had left, what a beautiful world this would be if we all could be like Angie.

Rest in peace Angela,

All our love,

Bill and Rose Booth

We remember Angie as a lovely neighbour who always had a smile and a word despite all the problems she was facing herself. She had a laugh which was infectious. She was a lovely, lovely lady.

From neighbours, Ken and Hilda Haigh.

Acknowledgements

I would like to thank the following people for all their help with putting this book together:

My co-author Lynne Barrett-Lee for her ability to put my memories and emotions into words; my editors, Carly and Briony, and all the team at Simon & Schuster; and my agent Andrew Lownie.

I would also like to thank the following people for their love and support given to myself, Angie, and our children:

First, our families who were there for us every step of the way, especially my brother Malcolm and his wife Eileen; Teresa Clark and all the staff at Milefield Primary School, for the support given to our children; Lynne Handley, thanks from the bottom of my heart for the support given to Angie and me through our two-year battle with cancer (Lynne, you were our rock); the nurses on the chemotherapy ward, Barnsley District Hospital (you lot really are angels on earth); last, but by no means least, my wonderful wife Angie for those thirty-five wonderful years you brought into my life.

In loving memory of Angela Rose Millthorpe, my parents Arthur and Daisy Millthorpe, my mother-in-law Winnie Yoxall and my dear cousin Anthony Booth.

God bless you all.